Yoga
Three in One

HB
HINKLER BOOKS

First published in 2006
by Hinkler Books Pty Ltd
45-55 Fairchild Street
Heatherton VIC 3202 Australia
www.hinklerbooks.com

Printed and bound in China

ISBN 10: 1 7415 7416 1
ISBN 13: 978 1 7415 7416 6

When practising Yoga, always do the warm up exercises before attempting
any individual postures. It is recommended that you check with your doctor
or healthcare professional before commencing any exercise regime. Whilst
every care has been taken in the preparation of this material, the Publishers
and their respective employees or agents will not accept responsibility for
injury or damage occasioned to any person as a result of participation in
the activities described in this book.

S I M P L Y
YOGA

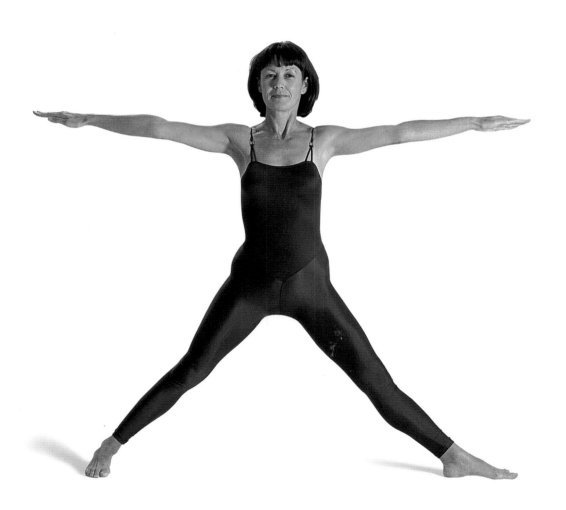

Creative Director: Sam Grimmer
Photography: Peter Wakeman

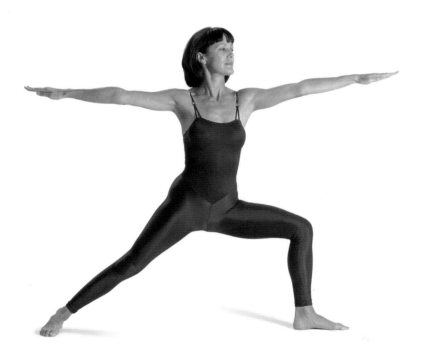

CONTENTS

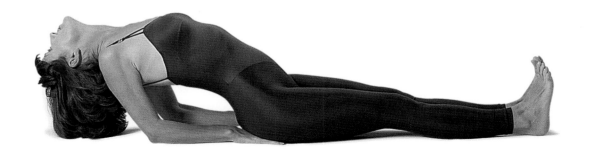

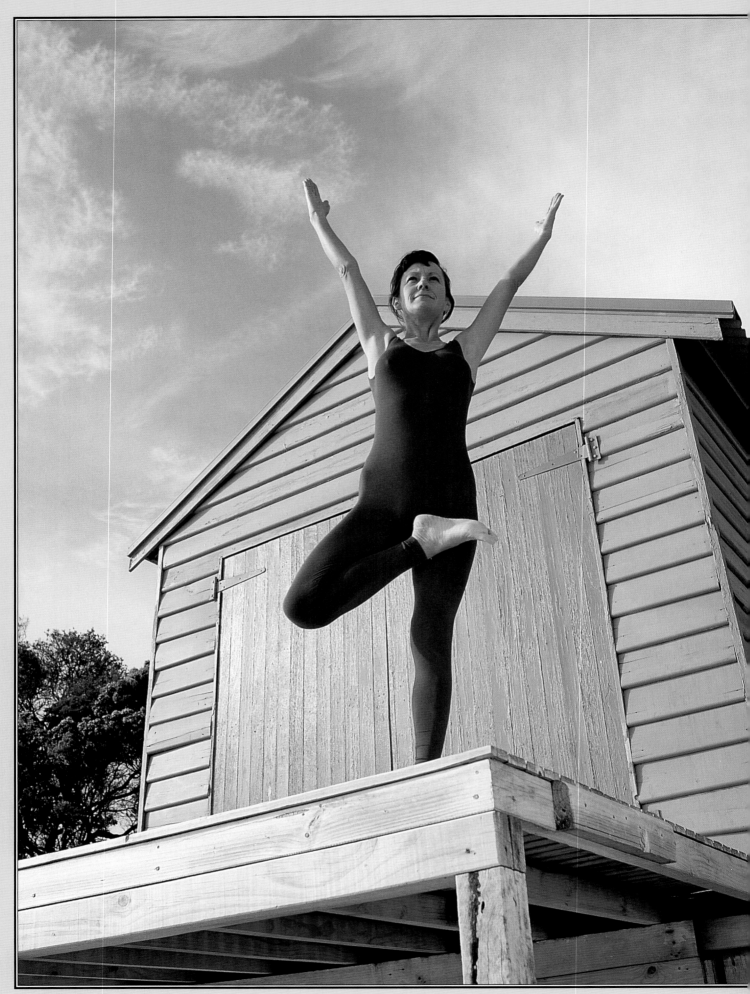

INTRODUCTION

This book is an easy guide to a balanced series of basic yoga postures. They are safe and effective for beginners and an excellent refresher course for the more experienced student.

The ancient science of yoga has been practised and passed on in the East for thousands of years, bringing health, happiness and peace of mind to those who have studied it. More recently, the benefits of yoga have been recognised and welcomed by the West and widely developed as a fitness regime. But the benefits are not merely physical. Yoga practitioners know that their quality of life improves on all levels – physical, emotional, mental and spiritual.

Here we are concerned with the physical aspects of yoga, but those of you who are able to practise the postures regularly will observe subtle and beautiful changes in other areas of your lives. Not only will your sense of physical wellbeing improve; feelings of stability, clarity and a greater capacity for concentration will emerge. Yoga can lift your capacity to succeed in all other areas of your life – your work, study, sport, and in your relationships with others.

It is recommended that you begin with the opening Savasana (corpse pose) with its yoga breathing routine, and proceed to the following postures. The sequence has been designed so each posture will flow smoothly on to the next, through a variety of kneeling, sitting, standing and lying down practices, returning again to the final Savasana and a beautiful relaxation practice.

As individuals vary in strength and flexibility, so the practice of yoga will be unique to each individual. Your body will tell you where you are strong and which areas need more practice. Do not be disheartened if you cannot reach the full extension of a posture as shown. Daily gentle practice will encourage your body to release its tensions. On some days a particular posture may seem more difficult while another may seem easier. This is normal. Be gentle and accommodating with yourself. A daily routine will encourage your body to respond to the movements. Most of all, have fun. Enjoy reaching for your full potential.

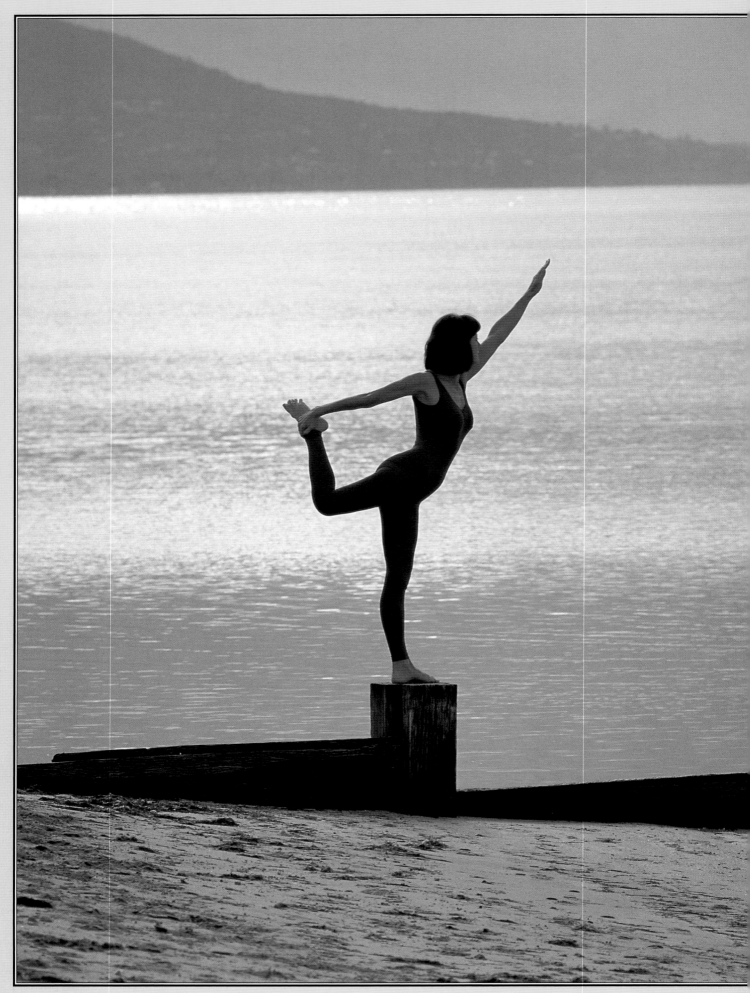

PRACTICAL MATTERS

It is important for you to follow the step-by-step directions and proceed at your own pace. As you do the postures, listen carefully to your body and recognise its warning signs. Rather than straining to achieve the required result, release your body gently into its own natural extensions. Do not try to push past pain. There is a difference between the feeling of stretching muscles and the pain associated with strain. If at any time you experience pain, slowly release out of the practice as you breathe out. Practised gently and regularly, the postures will increase your levels of fitness and flexibility.

A simple guide to the link between the breath and the body's movements during the postures: breathe in as the body stretches and expands; breathe out as the body contracts or folds forward. If there is no breathing instruction to follow, breathe normally.

Consult your health professional if you are in any doubt about your medical condition.

It is best to practise yoga when your stomach is empty. Before breakfast is ideal, or at least one hour before your evening meal.

REQUIREMENTS

A good yoga mat provides a soft non-slip surface. A rug or carpet are also suitable surfaces on which to practice.

Folded blankets and a small cushion are helpful for easing strain in certain postures. It is a recommended to cover yourself with a blanket when resting, to avoid feeling cold.

Practise in bare feet and wear appropriate, unrestrictive clothing or sportswear for ease of movement.

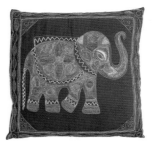

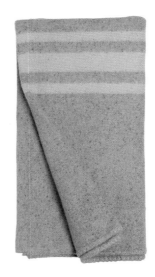

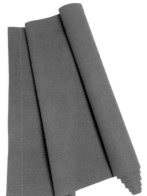

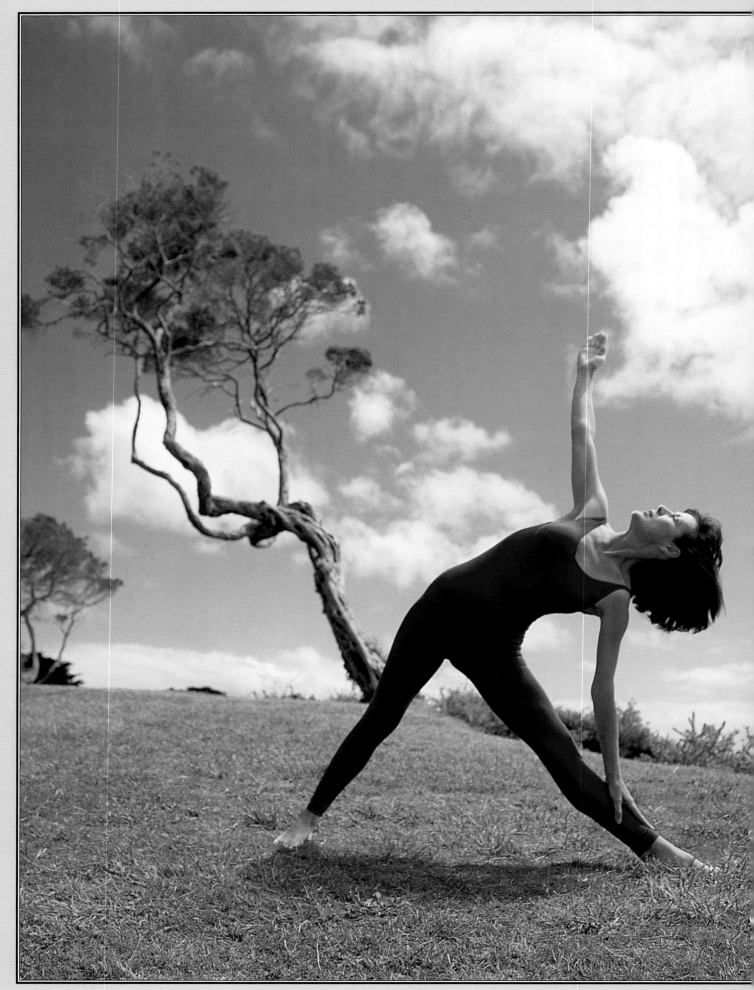

YOGA BREATHING

PRANAYAMA *(**Prana** - breath/life force **Yama** - natural law)*

Yoga breathing (Pranayama) is consciously observing the breath as we breathe in (inhale) and breathe out (exhale).

When the body is relaxed, the lungs are able to inhale and exhale more deeply. And the more deeply we exhale, the greater is our capacity to inhale fresh, clean air.

You will notice that yoga breathing involves breathing more deeply than your usual involuntary breathing. This deeper breathing brings more oxygen into your system. You may feel a little light-headed or dizzy when you begin. If you feel this happening at any time while doing the yoga postures (asanas), just take a moment to rest in the Child's Pose (Balasana).

The yoga breathing will change your usual pattern of breathing and will in turn change your state of mind. As your mind becomes clearer and more focused, your attention span will increase.

By beginning your yoga practice with a breathing sequence, you are increasing your mind's capacity to focus attention on the postures. As you follow the postures, continue to be aware of your breath.

There are many sequences of yoga breathing, but we have chosen Lobular Breathing as the ideal beginning to our simple posture sequence.

Lobular Breathing means breathing fully into the lobes of the lungs. We will breathe into the lower lobe (abdomen), the middle lobe (lower rib cage or diaphragm) and the upper lobe (top of the chest – just below the throat).

Yoga breathing is often practised in either the cross-legged pose (Sukasana) or the lotus pose (Padmasana). It can also be practised lying on the back in the relaxation pose (Savasana), and this is the way we will approach the breathing at the beginning of our practice.

So let our practice begin ...

CORPSE POSE

SAVASANA

Before you begin your practice it is important to let go of the outside world, to focus your mind and body in preparation for the practices that follow.

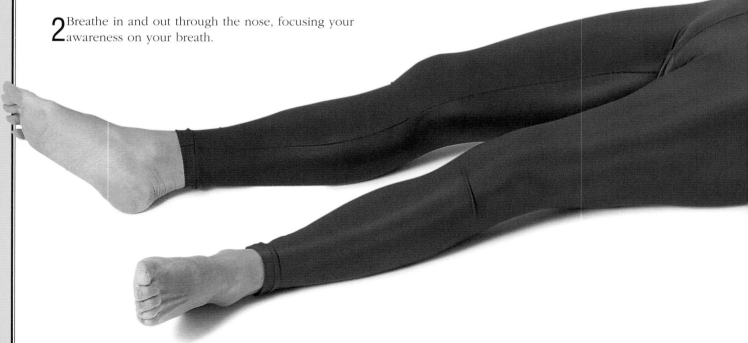

1 Lying on your back, relax your legs and allow your feet to fall outward. Relax your arms, turning the hands so the palms face upwards. Gently elongate your neck and allow the chin to tuck in slightly. Soften your face and close your eyes.

2 Breathe in and out through the nose, focusing your awareness on your breath.

3 Notice how you are feeling. Become aware of any tension, and as you breathe out, imagine the tension flowing out with the breath. As you breathe in, feel yourself filling up with positive, healing energy.

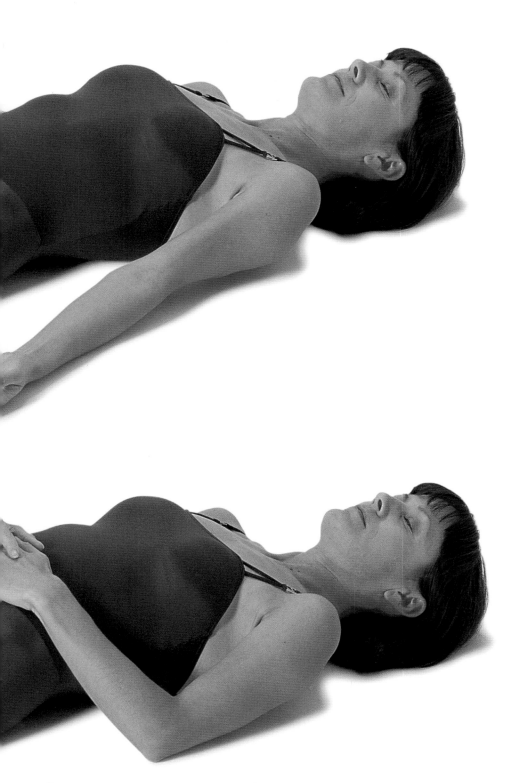

Breathing into the Abdomen

4 Gently place your hands one over the other, palms down, on your abdomen. Exhale slowly and completely. Then inhale, breathing into the abdomen, using the position of your hands to guide your breath. Allow the abdomen to rise and fill like a balloon. Hold your breath in momentarily, then slowly exhale. Hold without breath for a moment, then inhale again ... without rushing. Enjoy the feeling and the wonder of the breath. Breathe into the abdomen up to 5 times.

CORPSE POSE

SAVASANA *(continued)*

BREATHING INTO THE LOWER RIB CAGE (DIAPHRAGM)

5 Place your hands at the base of the rib cage and exhale slowly and completely. As you inhale, breathe into the lower rib cage and feel the lower ribs expanding. Hold the breath in momentarily, then slowly exhale and feel the lower ribs contract again. Hold without breath for a moment before inhaling again. Breathe into the lower ribs up to 5 times.

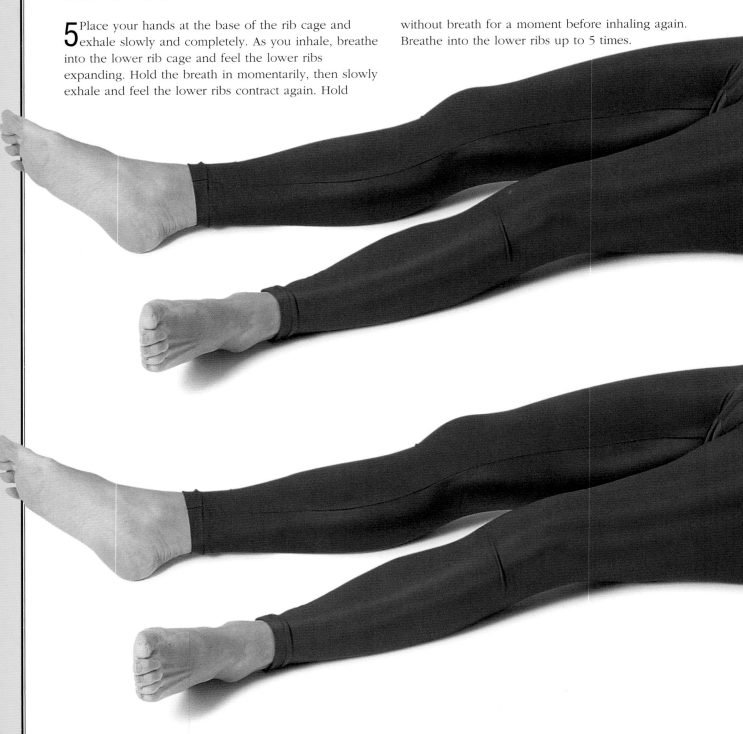

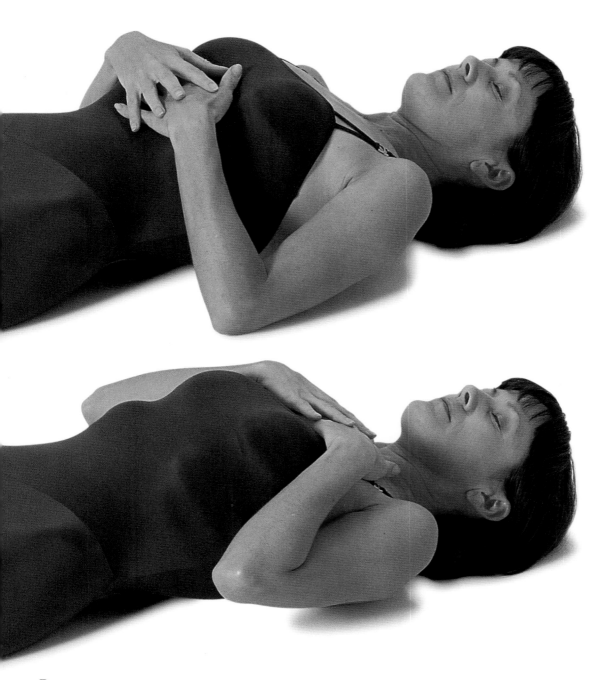

BREATHING INTO THE UPPER CHEST

6 Place the hands on the upper chest, below the throat. Exhale slowly and completely, then as you inhale, breathe slowly into the upper chest. This will feel a much deeper, fuller breath and you will feel expansion through the entire upper rib cage, front and back. Hold the breath for a moment before exhaling slowly and completely. Hold without breath for a moment, before inhaling again. Breathe into the upper chest up to 5 times.

Now relax and take one or two normal breaths.

LIMBERING

Gentle exercises to prepare the body for the stronger postures that follow.

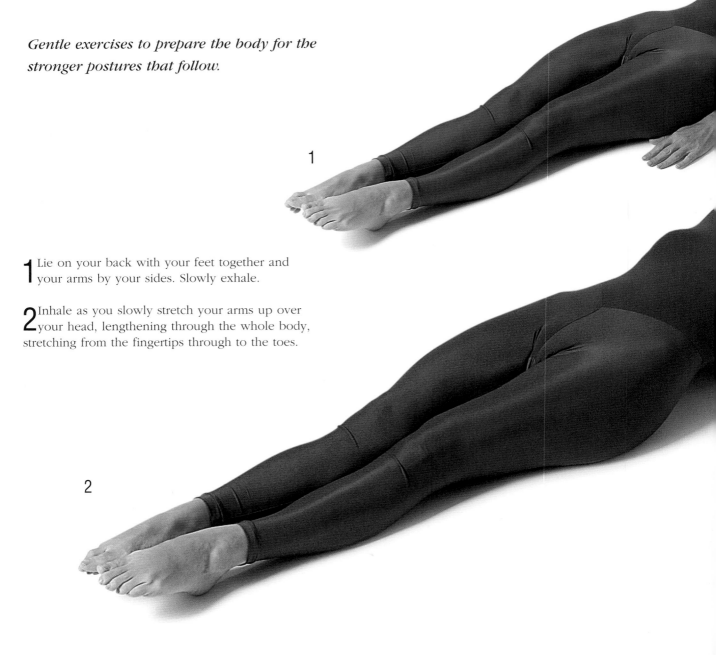

1

2

1 Lie on your back with your feet together and your arms by your sides. Slowly exhale.

2 Inhale as you slowly stretch your arms up over your head, lengthening through the whole body, stretching from the fingertips through to the toes.

3 Exhale as you lift your arms up to the ceiling and down to your sides again.

4 Inhale as you draw your right knee towards your chest and place your hands around your knee. Exhale as you lift your head towards your knee, tucking your chin into your chest, and hold for a moment. Then release the knee and lower your head to the floor.

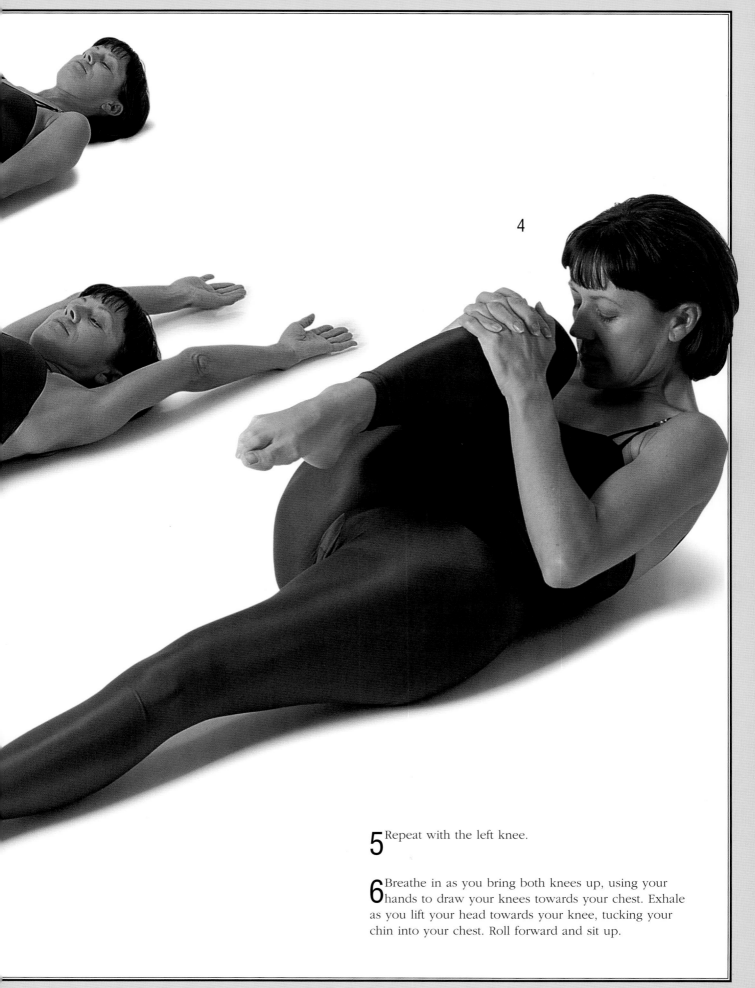

4

5 Repeat with the left knee.

6 Breathe in as you bring both knees up, using your hands to draw your knees towards your chest. Exhale as you lift your head towards your knee, tucking your chin into your chest. Roll forward and sit up.

HERO'S POSE

UTTHITA VIRASANA

A kneeling stretch, this posture opens the shoulders and gives a full stretch to the spine.

1 Kneel on the floor, with knees together and the feet tucked under the buttocks. Rest the hands on the thighs. Tuck your chin in slightly. Open your chest, and feel your spine lengthening from the tail bone to the crown of the head.

2 Inhale and stretch your arms forward and continue the stretch till your arms are above your head.

3 Exhale as you bend forward and rest your forehead on the floor. Stretch your arms straight along the floor in front of you. Try to keep the buttocks down on the heels.

4 Hold this position for up to 5 breaths. Each time you breathe in draw the rib cage forward over the thighs. As you breathe out, lengthen the stretch from the fingertips to the tail bone.

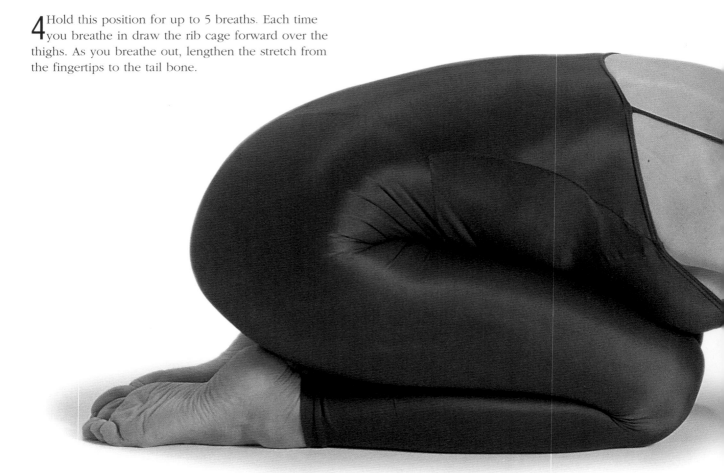

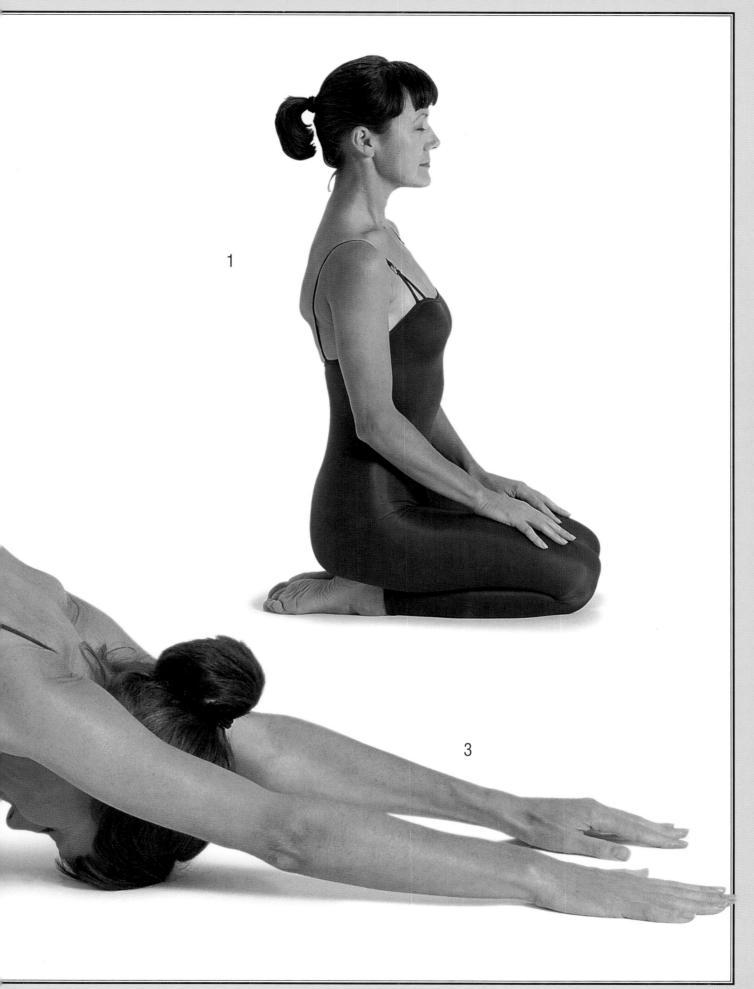

1

3

CAT STRETCH

Giving a rhythmical spinal stretch, the cat stretch strengthens the shoulders, wrists, spine and hip joints.

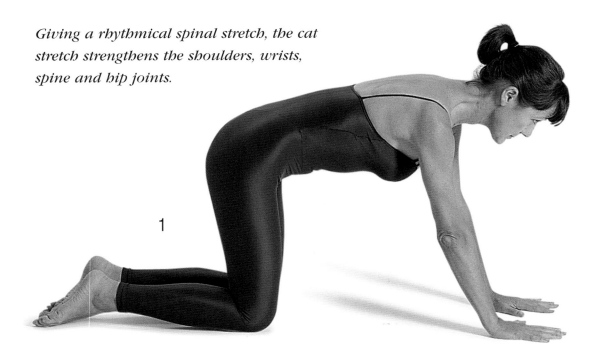

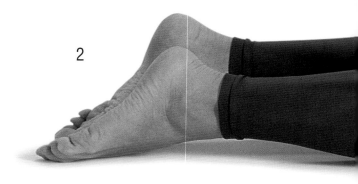

1 Begin this practice on your hands and knees, with your shoulders directly above your hands, and your hips directly above your knees.

2 Inhale as you roll your shoulders back and tilt your pelvis back and up. Tilt the chin and look up as the back concaves.

3 Exhale as you reverse the posture. Draw the abdomen in, squeezing all the breath out of it, as you arch your back. Tuck your chin into your chest and look down at your feet.

4 Continue concaving the back (inhaling) and arching the back (exhaling) gently and evenly, up to 5 times.

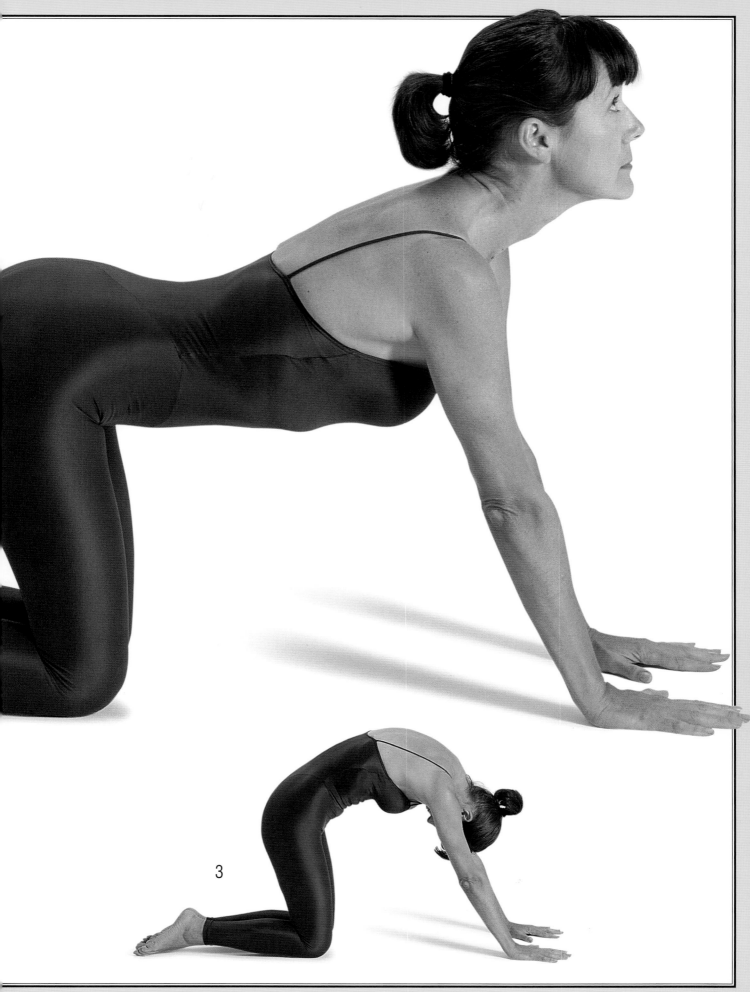

3

CHILD'S POSE

BALASANA

This is a beautiful resting pose. It relaxes the back, the shoulders and the arms.

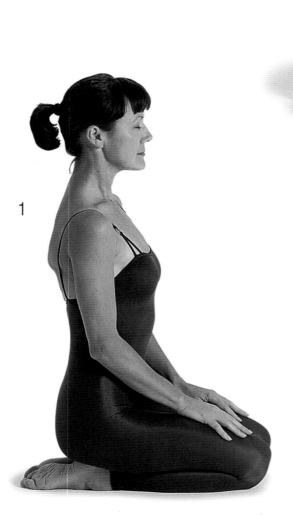

1

1 Kneel on the floor with your heels under your buttocks. Bend your torso forward so that your abdomen and chest are resting on your thighs. Tuck your chin under and allow your forehead to touch the floor. Bring your arms back so that they lie alongside the body, hands palm upward beside the feet. Soften the shoulders and the arms.

2 Bring your awareness to your breath. Breathe into any feelings of tightness. Let go of any tension with the exhaling breath. Rest in this pose before moving to the next posture.

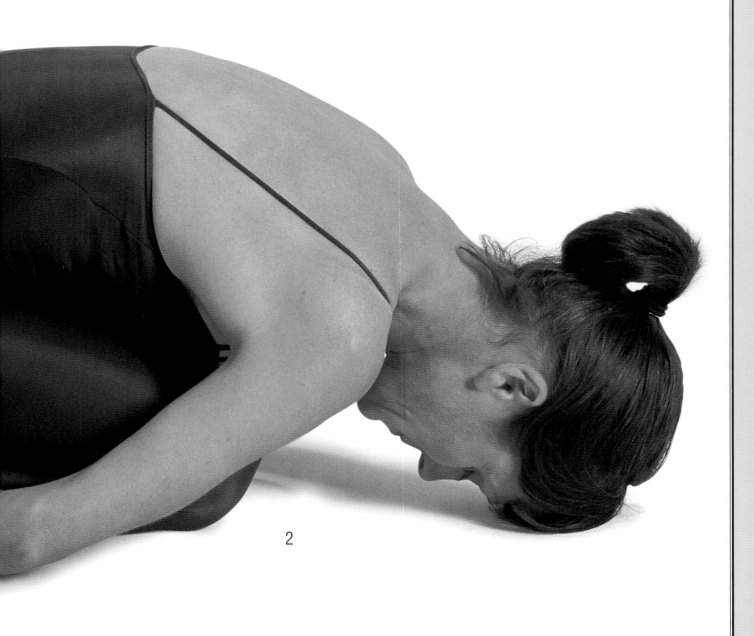

2

SOFTER

Kneel on the floor with your heels under your buttocks. Lean forward and rest your elbows on the floor a little further apart than your knees. Making fists of your hands, place one fist on top of the other. Rest your forehead on your fists. Follow direction no 2 above.

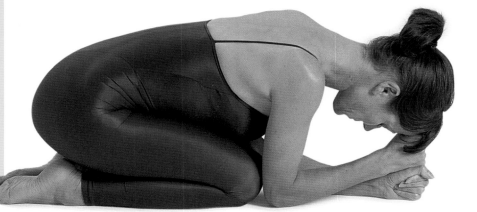

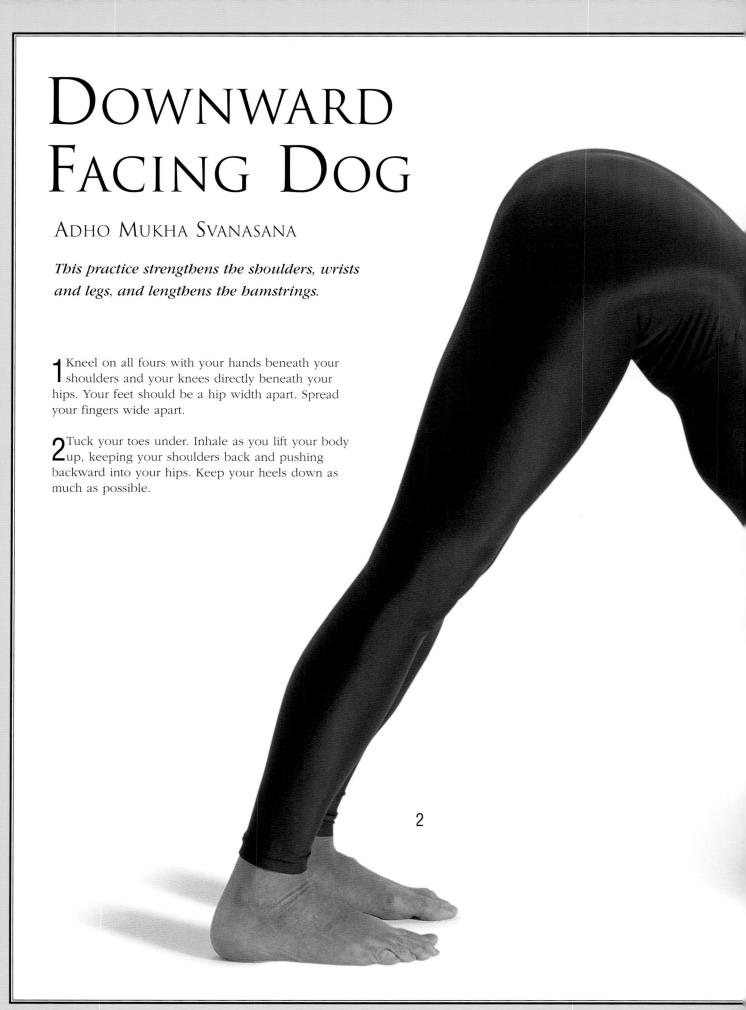

DOWNWARD FACING DOG

ADHO MUKHA SVANASANA

This practice strengthens the shoulders, wrists and legs, and lengthens the hamstrings.

1 Kneel on all fours with your hands beneath your shoulders and your knees directly beneath your hips. Your feet should be a hip width apart. Spread your fingers wide apart.

2 Tuck your toes under. Inhale as you lift your body up, keeping your shoulders back and pushing backward into your hips. Keep your heels down as much as possible.

2

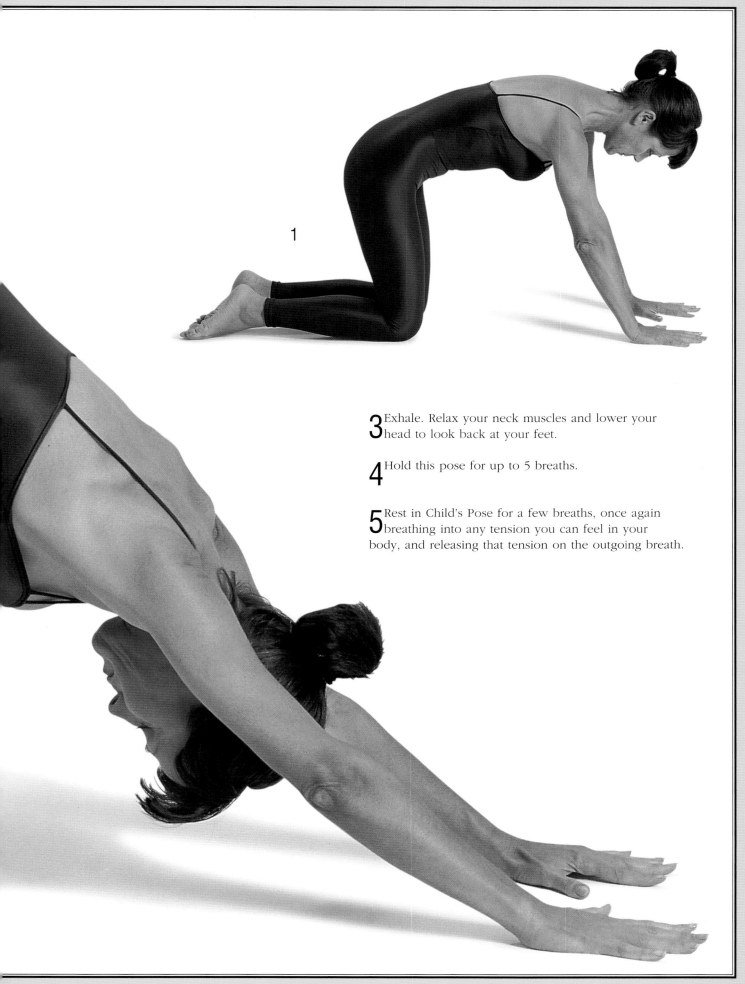

1

3 Exhale. Relax your neck muscles and lower your head to look back at your feet.

4 Hold this pose for up to 5 breaths.

5 Rest in Child's Pose for a few breaths, once again breathing into any tension you can feel in your body, and releasing that tension on the outgoing breath.

THE COBRA

BHUJANGASANA

This pose arches the back like the curve of a snake, toning and strengthening the vertebral muscles.

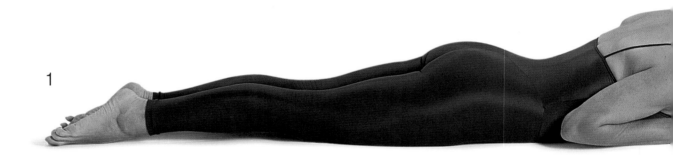

1

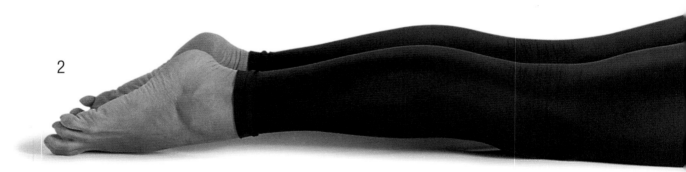

2

1 Lie on your front with your arms outstretched and your forehead touching the mat. Bring your arms back towards your body until your hands are directly beneath your shoulders. Keep your elbows tucked in beside the body.

2 As you inhale, lift your chin, your neck and then your chest, curving your spine up and back. Press down on the mat with your hands, gently increasing the arch in your back. Try to keep your feet together. Hold for 5 breaths.

3 Exhale as you release down in the reverse order – lowering your chest first, then your chin, then curve your head down till your forehead is once again on the mat.

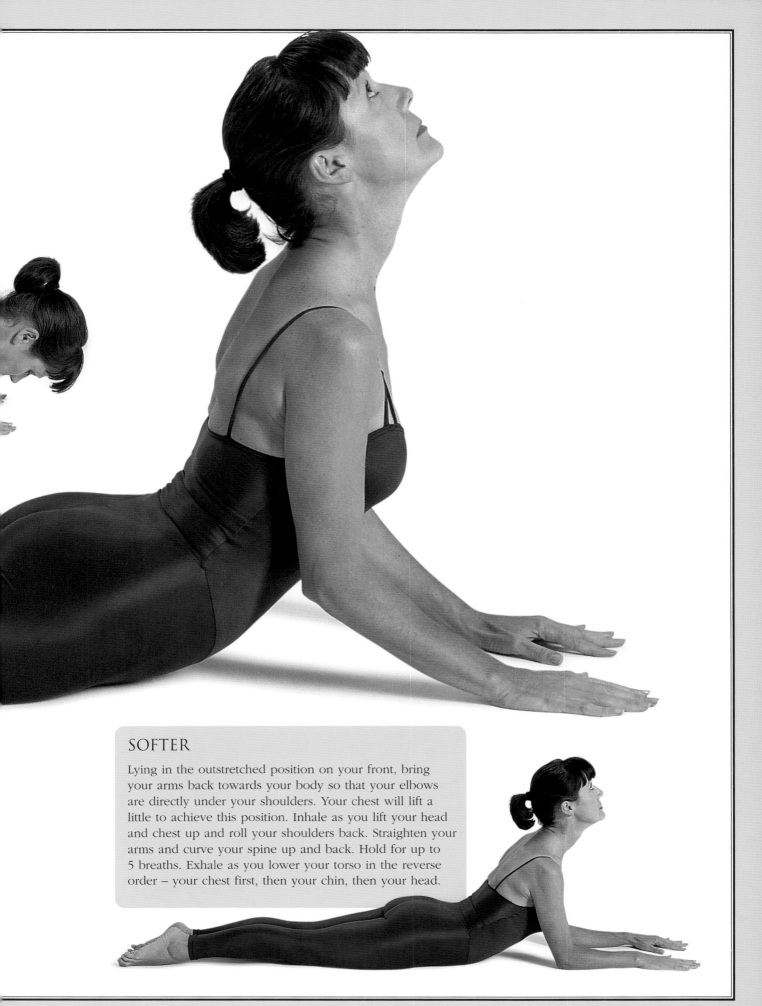

SOFTER

Lying in the outstretched position on your front, bring your arms back towards your body so that your elbows are directly under your shoulders. Your chest will lift a little to achieve this position. Inhale as you lift your head and chest up and roll your shoulders back. Straighten your arms and curve your spine up and back. Hold for up to 5 breaths. Exhale as you lower your torso in the reverse order – your chest first, then your chin, then your head.

STANDING FORWARD BEND

UTTANASANSA

This restful practice loosens the neck and shoulder muscles, extends the spine and strengthens the leg muscles.

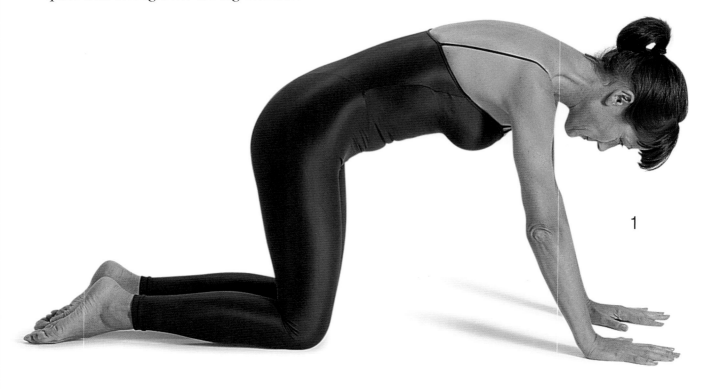

1

1 From the cobra pose, raise your body to the all-fours position and walk your knees in towards your hands.

2 Spread your fingers on the floor and tuck your toes under. Walk your hands back towards your knees.

3 Standing on your feet now, allow your head to continue to hang forward. Place your hands around your elbows.

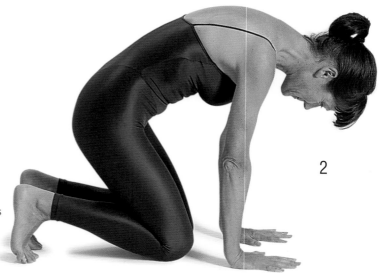

2

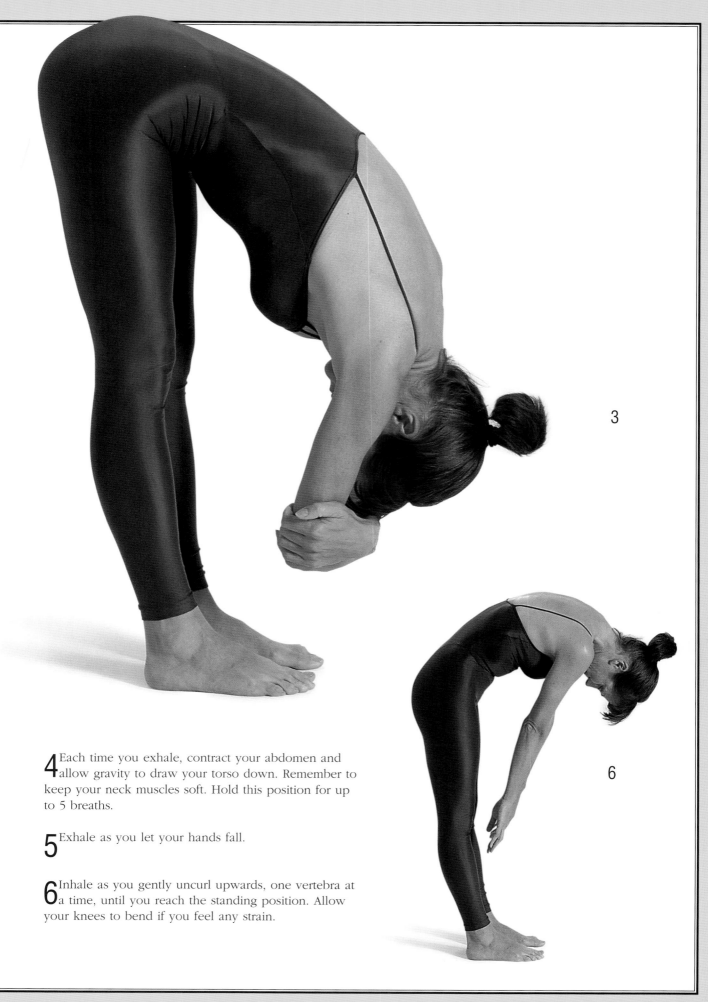

3

4 Each time you exhale, contract your abdomen and allow gravity to draw your torso down. Remember to keep your neck muscles soft. Hold this position for up to 5 breaths.

5 Exhale as you let your hands fall.

6 Inhale as you gently uncurl upwards, one vertebra at a time, until you reach the standing position. Allow your knees to bend if you feel any strain.

6

SHOULDER ROTATIONS

For releasing any tightness in the neck and shoulders.

1 Stand with your feet a hip width apart and your arms hanging relaxed by your sides.

2 Inhale as you bring your shoulders up to your ears. Roll your shoulders firmly back. Squeeze them as close together as you can. Then exhale as you roll them downward and return to the starting position.

3 Inhale as you squeeze your shoulders together behind you. Bring them up to your ears, and exhale as you roll them forward and down.

4 Continue rotating your shoulders up to 5 times forwards and backwards.

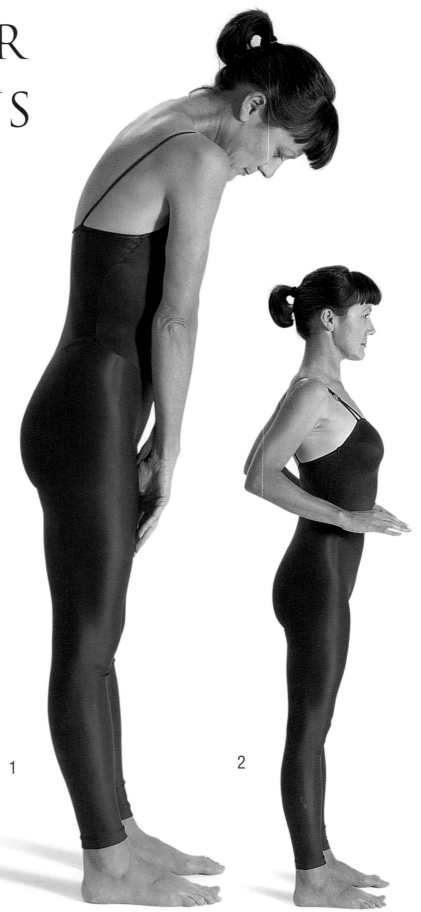

1

2

MOUNTAIN POSE

TADASANA

This simple pose encourages balance, good posture, elongation of the spine, and vertebral alignment.

1 Stand with your feet together, your arms relaxed by your sides and your weight evenly balanced over the feet. Keep your chest open. Look straight ahead and soften your gaze.

2 Gently 'lift' the knee and thigh muscles, tuck your tail bone under and abdomen in. Feel your spine lengthen from the tail bone to the crown of your head. Allow the back of your head to lift slightly and tuck your chin in.

3 Remain steady but continue to 'lift' and stand tall. Hold for up to 5 breaths.

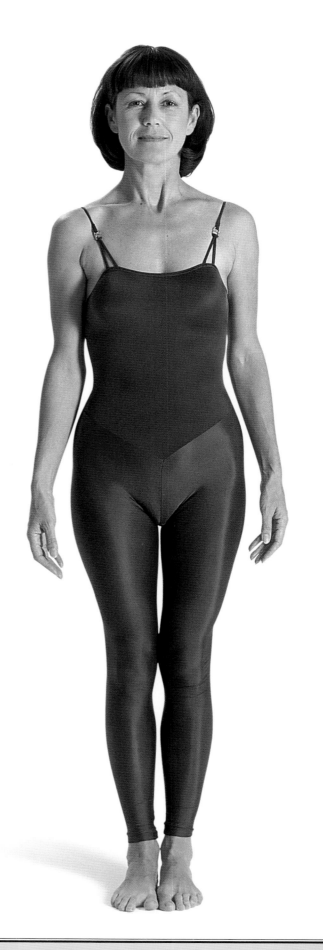

CHAIR POSE

UTKATASANA

A standing posture that strengthens the shins, knees, thighs and hips.

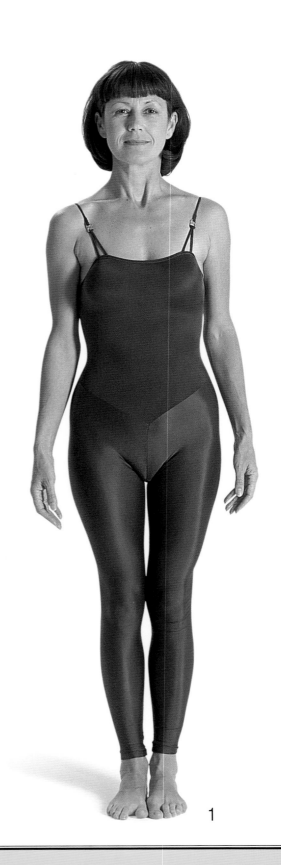

1 Stand with your feet together in the Mountain Pose, keeping your back tall and straight.

2 Lift your arms straight above your head. Your upper arms should be directly beside your ears. Tuck your chin in slightly. Place your hands in the prayer position with the thumbs locked.

3 Tucking your tailbone under, exhale as you squat as if to sit on a chair.

4 Hold for up to 5 breaths. On each outward breath, sink a little deeper while maintaining the upward stretch.

5 Inhale as you straighten your legs and return to the standing position.

SOFTER

As you exhale, sink into the 'sitting' position, and as you inhale, straighten your legs to the standing position. Do this up to 5 times.

1

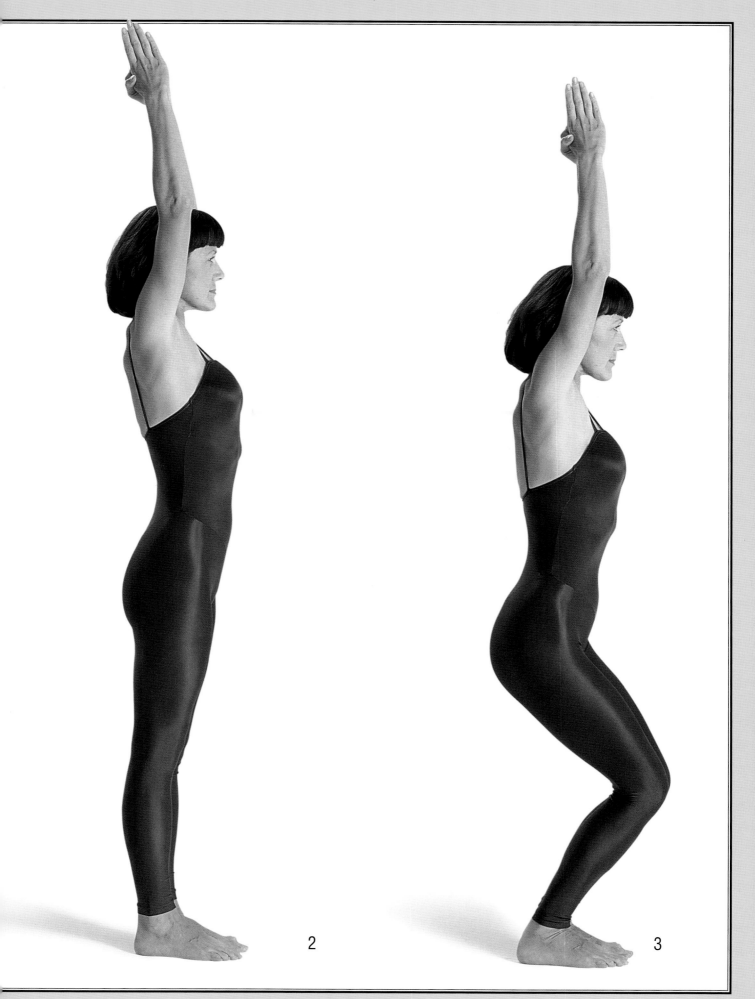

2

3

TRIANGLE POSE

TRIKONASANA

This is a strong posture for opening and stretching the shoulders. It will also tone the back, the hips and the inner thighs.

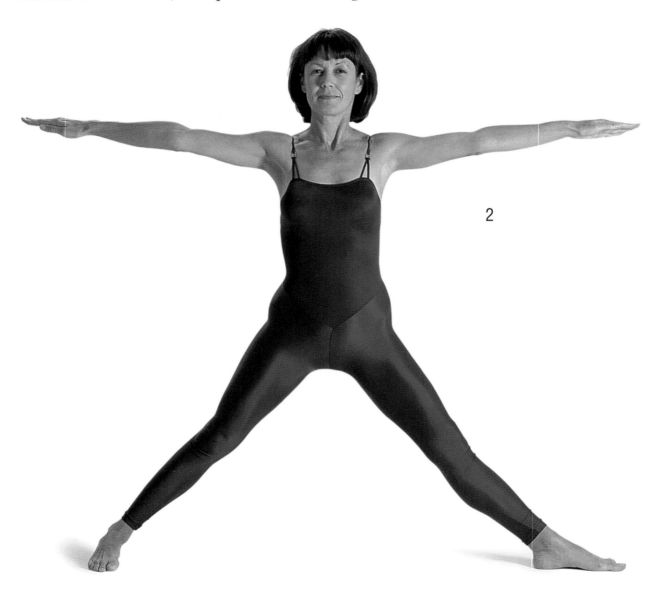

2

1 Stand with your feet a little more than 1 metre (3 ft) apart. Point your right foot straight ahead. Turn your left foot at right angles to it, to the left.

2 Inhale and stretch both arms out to the sides at shoulder level with the palms facing downward. Roll your shoulders back. Exhale.

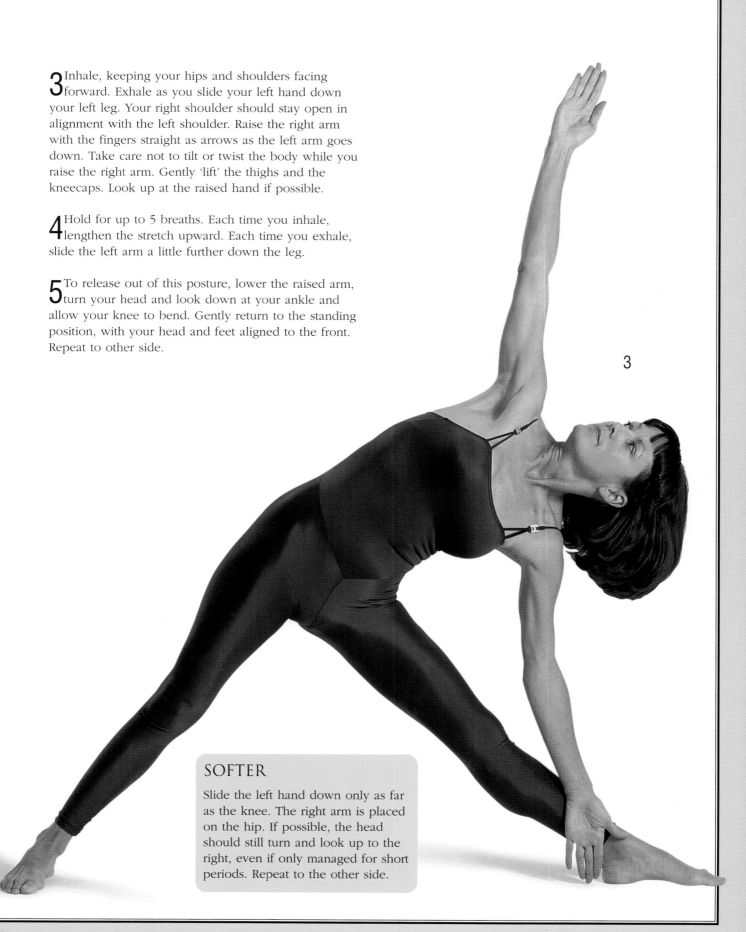

3 Inhale, keeping your hips and shoulders facing forward. Exhale as you slide your left hand down your left leg. Your right shoulder should stay open in alignment with the left shoulder. Raise the right arm with the fingers straight as arrows as the left arm goes down. Take care not to tilt or twist the body while you raise the right arm. Gently 'lift' the thighs and the kneecaps. Look up at the raised hand if possible.

4 Hold for up to 5 breaths. Each time you inhale, lengthen the stretch upward. Each time you exhale, slide the left arm a little further down the leg.

5 To release out of this posture, lower the raised arm, turn your head and look down at your ankle and allow your knee to bend. Gently return to the standing position, with your head and feet aligned to the front. Repeat to other side.

3

SOFTER

Slide the left hand down only as far as the knee. The right arm is placed on the hip. If possible, the head should still turn and look up to the right, even if only managed for short periods. Repeat to the other side.

WARRIOR POSE

VIRABHADRASANA

This strengthening practice opens the hips and the shoulders, tones the arms, lower back, thighs and knees.

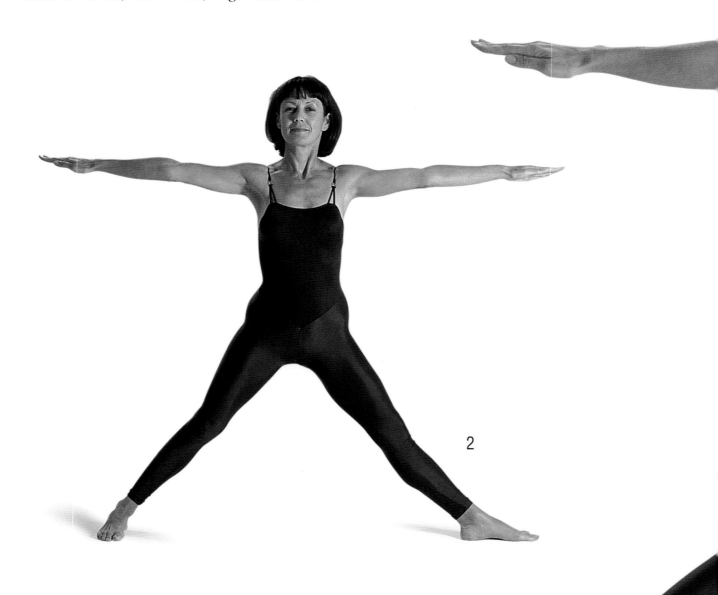

2

1 Standing with your feet a little more than 1 metre (3 ft) apart, point your right foot to the front and your left foot at right angles to it, to the left.

2 As you breathe in, raise your arms to shoulder level with the palms facing down and fingers pointed like arrows.

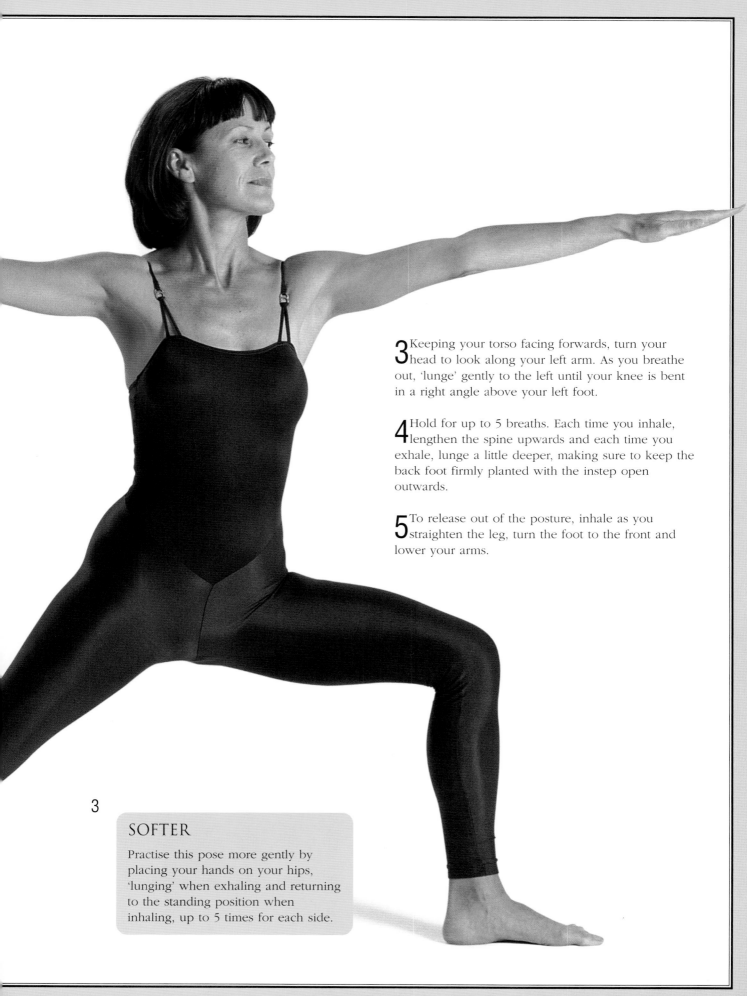

3 Keeping your torso facing forwards, turn your head to look along your left arm. As you breathe out, 'lunge' gently to the left until your knee is bent in a right angle above your left foot.

4 Hold for up to 5 breaths. Each time you inhale, lengthen the spine upwards and each time you exhale, lunge a little deeper, making sure to keep the back foot firmly planted with the instep open outwards.

5 To release out of the posture, inhale as you straighten the leg, turn the foot to the front and lower your arms.

3

SOFTER

Practise this pose more gently by placing your hands on your hips, 'lunging' when exhaling and returning to the standing position when inhaling, up to 5 times for each side.

Dancer's Pose

Natarajasana

A balancing posture that focuses the mind, the body and the breath. It works particularly to strengthen the shoulders, lower back, thighs, the flexors and the legs.

1 Stand with your feet together and your arms by your sides in the Mountain Pose (Tadasana).

2 Bend the right knee, lifting the foot up behind you. Exhale and take hold of your ankle with your right hand. Squeeze the foot into the buttock.

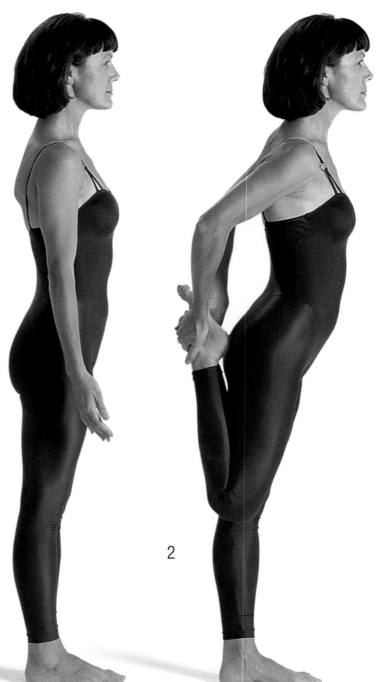

1

2

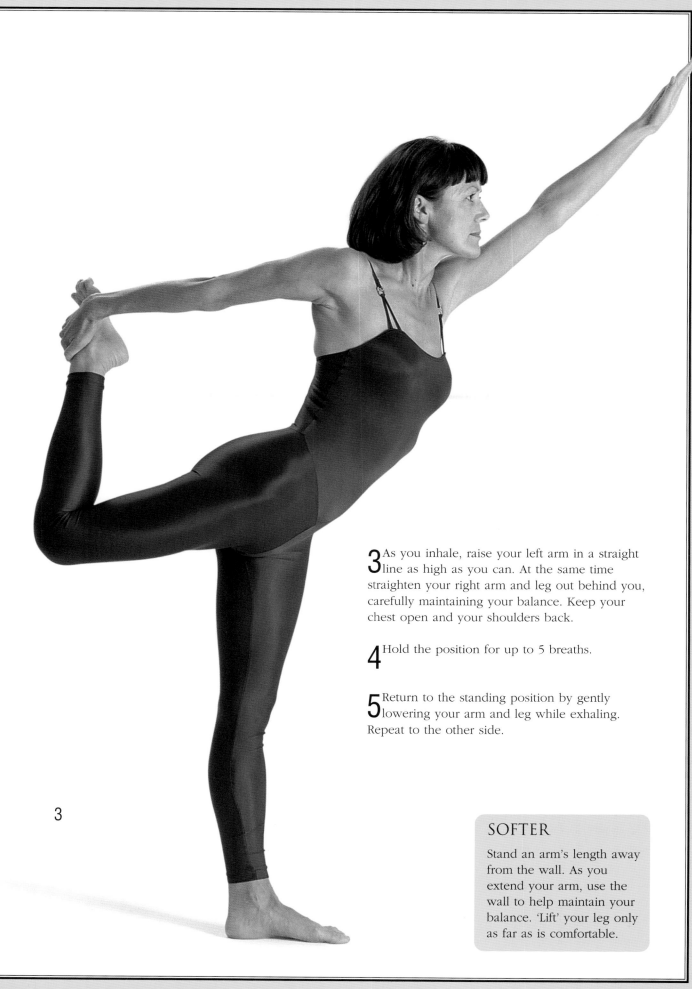

3 As you inhale, raise your left arm in a straight line as high as you can. At the same time straighten your right arm and leg out behind you, carefully maintaining your balance. Keep your chest open and your shoulders back.

4 Hold the position for up to 5 breaths.

5 Return to the standing position by gently lowering your arm and leg while exhaling. Repeat to the other side.

3

SOFTER

Stand an arm's length away from the wall. As you extend your arm, use the wall to help maintain your balance. 'Lift' your leg only as far as is comfortable.

BOUND ANGLE

BADDHA KONASANA

Stimulating circulation to the pelvic and reproductive organs, this sitting posture also tones the muscles in the back and releases the hips.

1 Sit with the feet drawn towards you and the soles of your feet together. Let your knees relax out and down as far as they will go.

2 Hold the toes by wrapping both hands around both feet. Lengthen your spine and straighten your arms. Allow the shoulders to relax down and back, and the chest to rise. Relax your hips and allow the soles of the feet to open.

3 Hold for up to 5 breaths. Soften and relax the hips each time you exhale.

4 Return to the starting position (knees drawn up and soles of the feet on the mat) as you gently exhale.

SOFTER

Sitting against the wall with a cushion to support your lower back, bring the soles of the feet together. Rest your hands on your knees. As you exhale, gently push down on your knees with your hands. Alternatively, lying on your back, draw the soles of your feet as far up to your groin as you can. Rest your hands on your thighs. On each exhalation allow your knees to drop down a little further towards the floor.

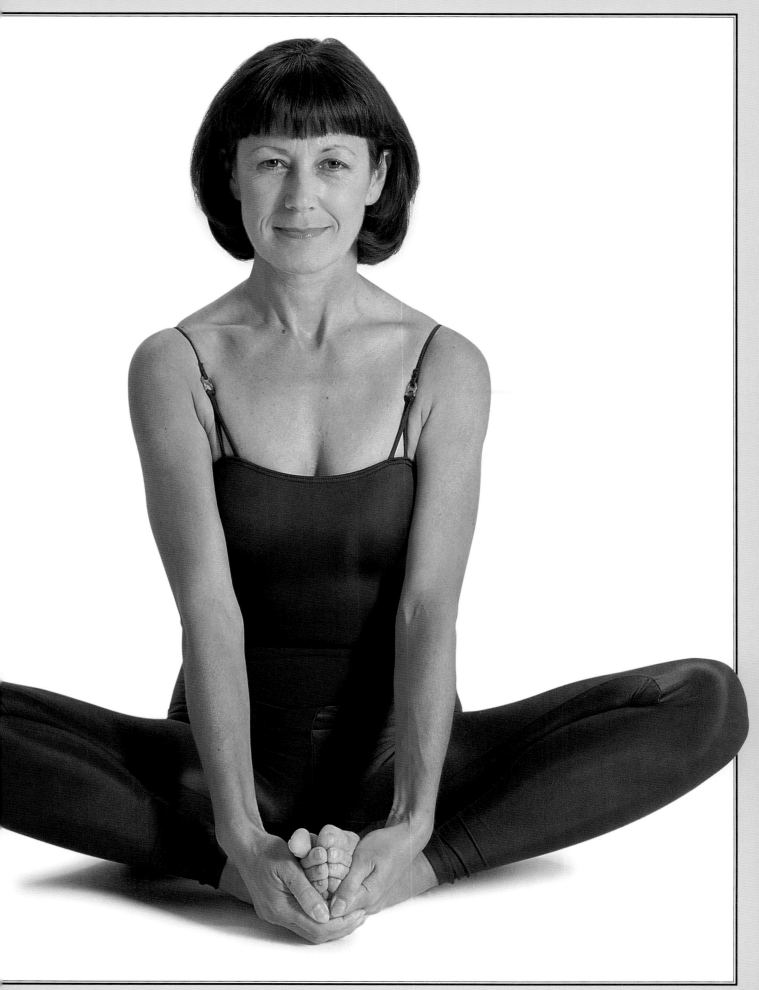

Half Bridge

Setu Bandha Sarvangasana

A strengthening and toning posture for the thighs, buttocks, and the lower and middle back.

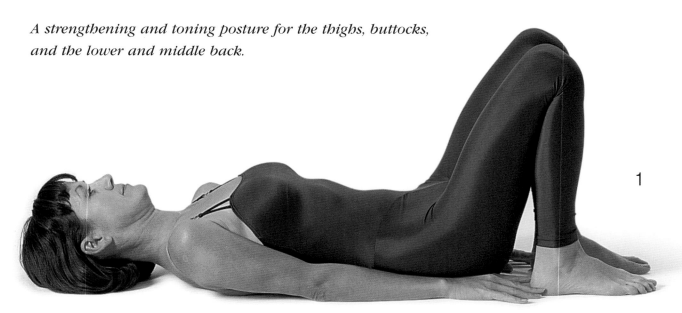

1

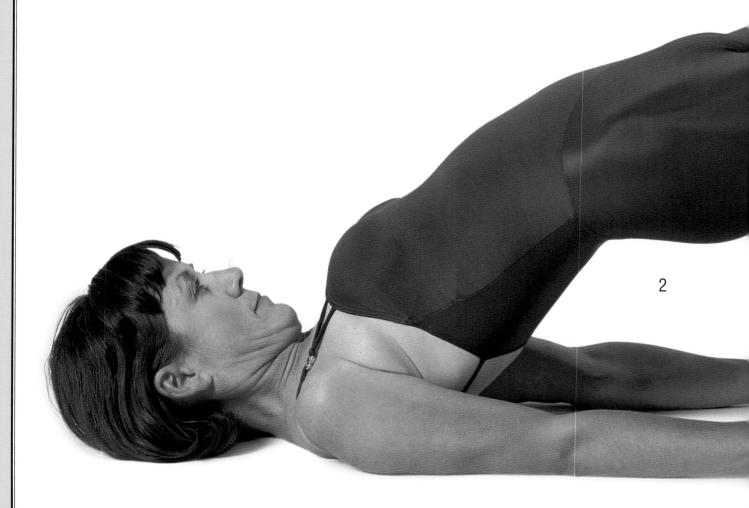

2

1 Lie flat on your back with arms at your sides. Tuck your chin in and lengthen your spine. Bend your knees and bring your feet up towards your buttocks as far as they will comfortably go. Keep your feet a hip width apart. Exhale completely.

2 Inhale as you push down on the floor with your feet, gently raising your hips, rolling your spine up slowly, one vertebra at a time. Lengthen your arms towards your ankles under your body, drawing the elbows and shoulders in.

3 Your head, neck and shoulders remain flat on the mat. Hold this position for up to 5 breaths.

4 Exhale as you lower your back one vertebra at a time.

SOFTER

Leaving your arms on the floor beside you, raise your hips and chest as you inhale. Pause for a moment, then exhale as you lower your torso back to the ground. Repeat up to 5 times.

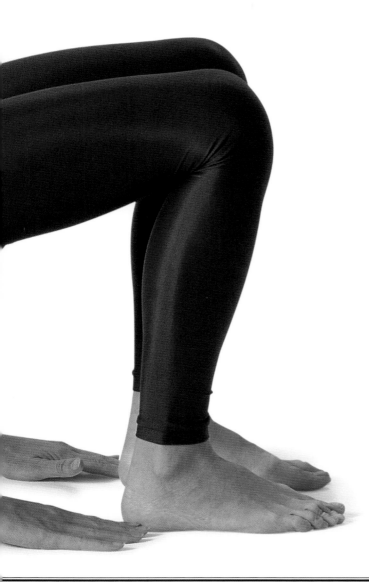

SHOULDER STAND

SARVANGASANA

This inverted pose stimulates blood circulation and increases the oxygen supply to the head. It also stimulates the thyroid gland, and strengthens the back and abdominal muscles.

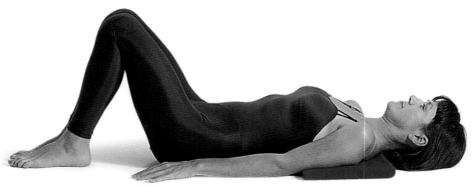

1

1 Lying on the floor with your legs and feet together and your arms by your sides, exhale completely.

2 Inhale as you draw your knees up to your chest and exhale as you continue to roll your knees up to your forehead. Place your hands as far up your back to your shoulder blades as you can.

3 Maintaining your balance, carefully extend your legs to the vertical position. Keep your eyes open and look up at your feet. Hold for up to 5 breaths.

4 To come down, exhale and gently bend your knees until they are touching your forehead again. Lower your hands to the floor and use them for support as you roll your torso down. Inhale as you straighten your legs along the mat.

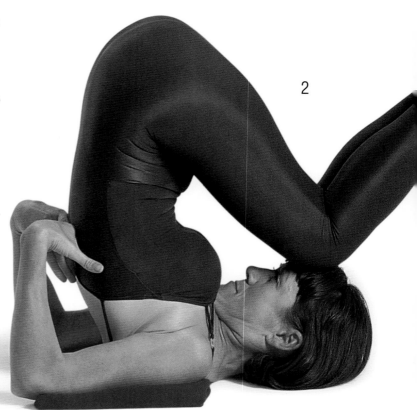

2

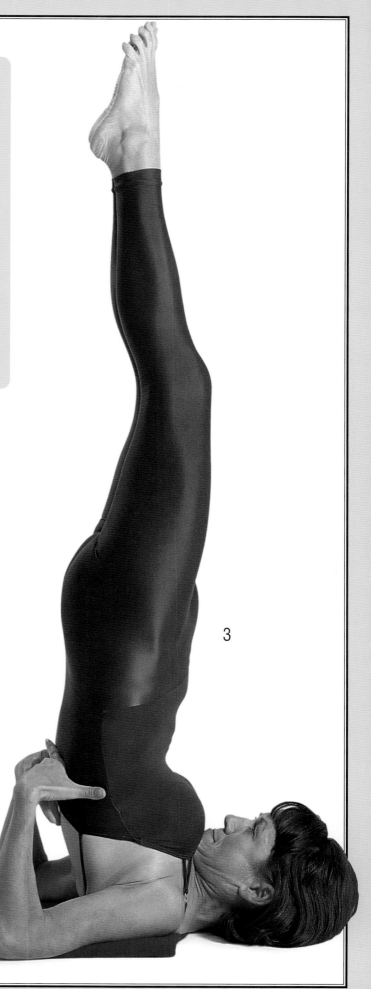

SOFTER

Using the wall to help you achieve the inverted pose

1 Lying on the floor, bring your hips close to the wall. Align your body so that your feet rest on the wall, slightly above the height of your bent knees. Your arms should be by your sides and your chin tucked in slightly. Exhale completely.

2 Inhale and push against the wall with your feet, raising your hips as high as you can. Place your hands in the small of your back, thumbs turned in towards the spine, and fingers pointing out around your hips. Exhale.

3 Breathe in and slowly walk your feet up the wall as far as you can. Hold in this position for up to 5 breaths. Breathe out and walk your feet gently down again.

3

FISH POSE

MATSYASANA

The fish pose is a lovely counter pose to the shoulder stand. It encourages good posture, opens the chest and strengthens the neck muscles.

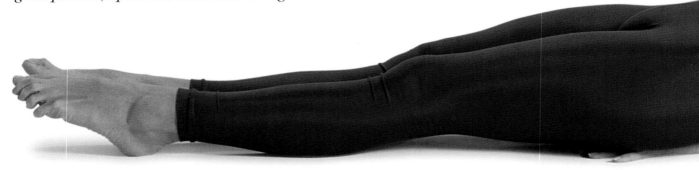

1 Lie flat on your back with your knees bent and your knees and feet together. Push down on the mat with your feet and lift your buttocks. Place your hands palms downward under your buttocks. The elbows should be tucked in under the back. Lower your buttocks onto your hands.

2 Exhale as you straighten your legs along the mat. As you inhale, push your elbows into the mat, and bend your arms so that your chest rises. Keep your legs and buttocks on the floor, and allow your head to drop gently back.

3 Breathe deeply and comfortably into the expanded chest for up to 5 breaths.

4 To come out of the posture, lift your head slightly, relax your elbows and breathe out as you lower your back to the floor.

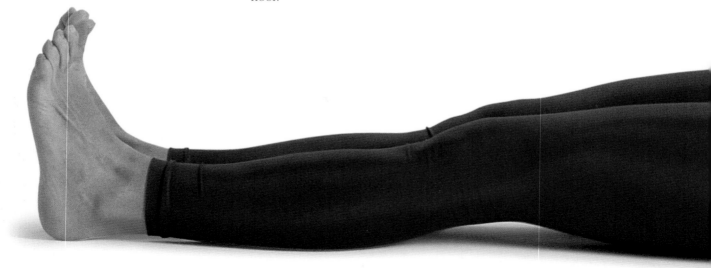

1

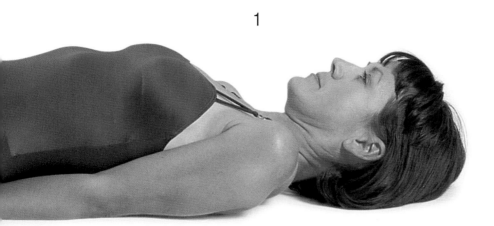

2

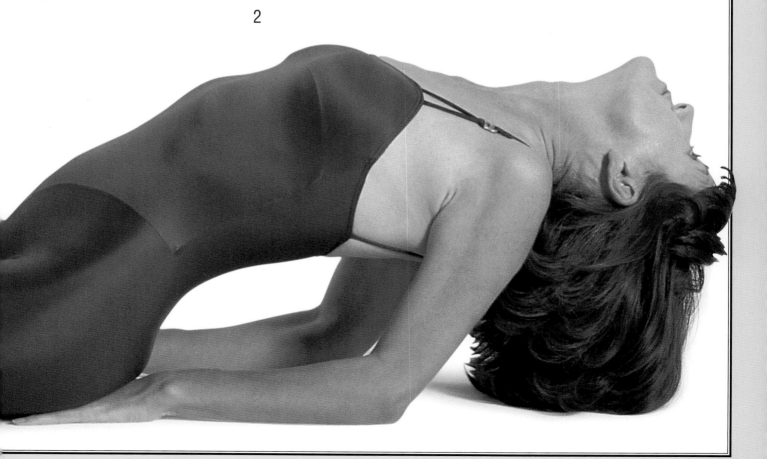

TWISTING POSE

MATSYENDRASANA

*For strengthening and toning the shoulders, spine and
buttocks, and massaging the internal organs.*

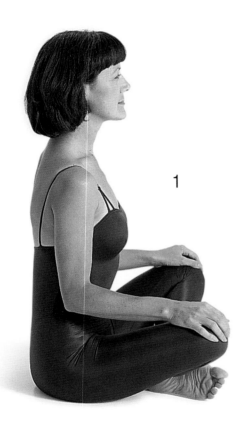

1

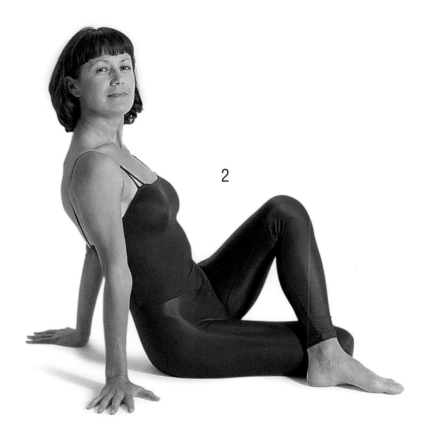

2

1 Sit with your legs crossed so that the left foot is
in front of the right. Push your sitting bones back
and lengthen your spine.

2 Exhale and bring your left foot over your
right knee.

3 Roll your left shoulder back and place your left
hand on the mat behind the buttocks at the base
of your spine. Hug your left knee with your right
arm. Hold the position for up to 5 breaths. On each
inbreath extend the spine upward. On every
outbreath, twist gently to look over your left shoulder.

4 Return to the sitting position with legs crossed.
Bend your torso forward over your crossed legs as
you exhale. As you inhale, straighten the torso again.

5 Change your leg position so that the right foot is
now in front of the left and repeat the
instructions twisting to the opposite side.

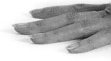

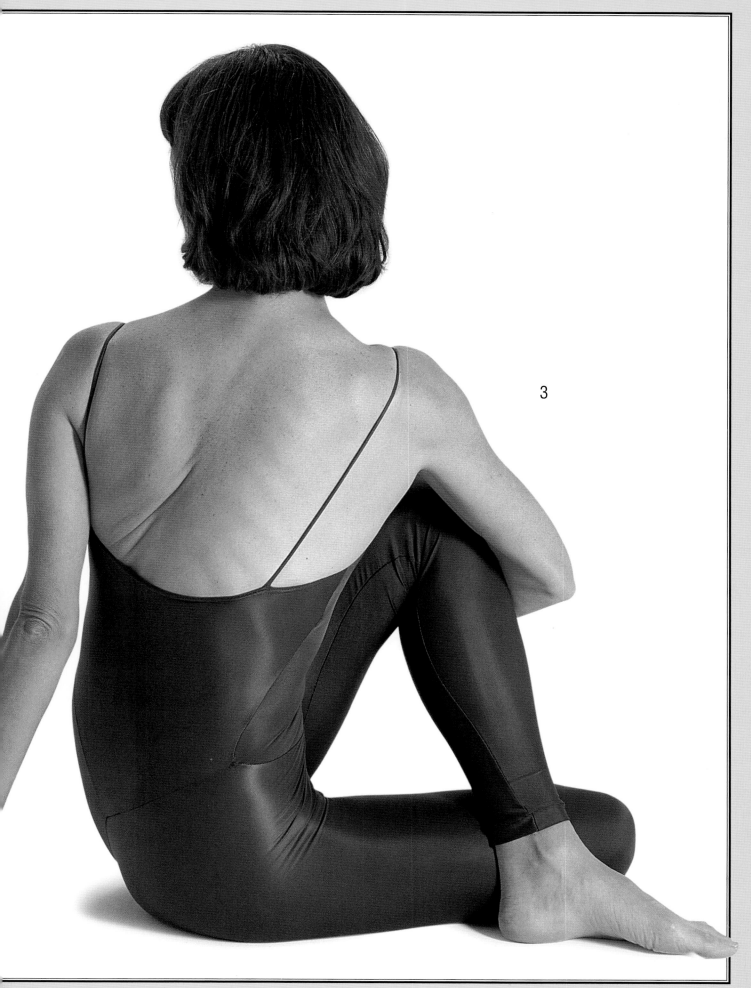

3

TWISTING II

A Softer Alternative

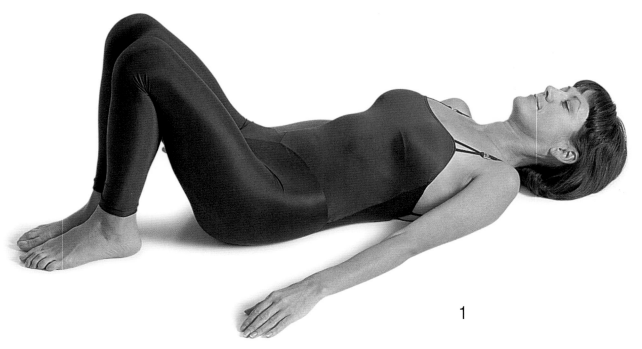

1

1 Lie on your back with your knees bent and your feet on the floor. Place your arms a little away from your sides with the palms facing down.

2 Lift the left leg and cross it over the right knee.

3 Exhale as you roll both legs to the right and roll your head gently to the left. It is important to keep your chin tucked in and both shoulders on the floor.

4 Hold the position for up to 5 breaths. Inhale as you roll back to the centre and uncross your legs. Repeat to the other side.

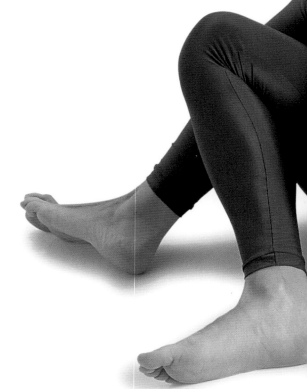

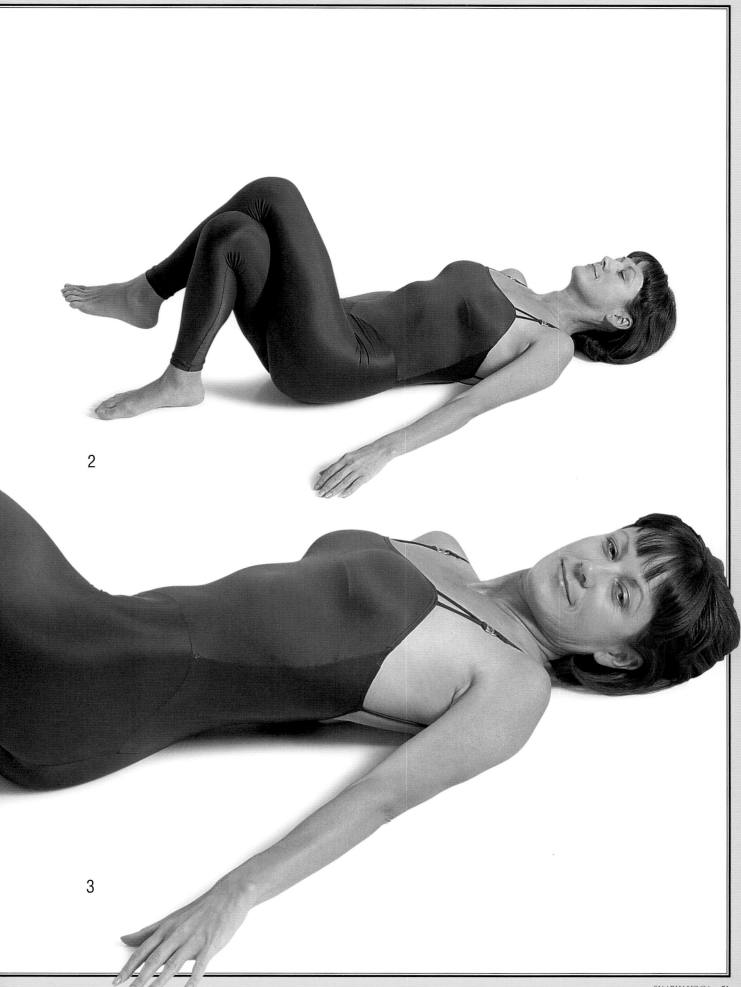

2

3

Hand to Foot

Ubhaya Padangusthasana

This pose works to open the back, lengthen the hamstrings and strengthen the shoulders. It is an excellent preparation for the corpse pose which follows it.

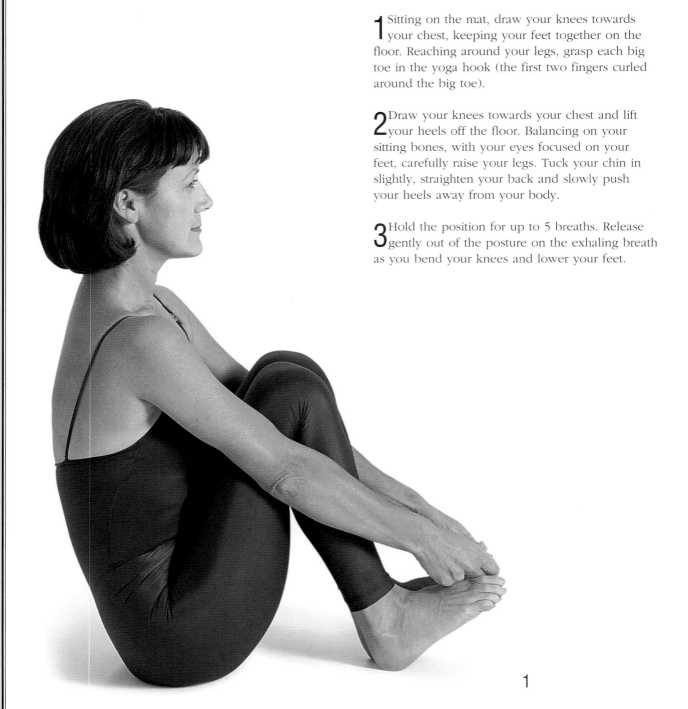

1 Sitting on the mat, draw your knees towards your chest, keeping your feet together on the floor. Reaching around your legs, grasp each big toe in the yoga hook (the first two fingers curled around the big toe).

2 Draw your knees towards your chest and lift your heels off the floor. Balancing on your sitting bones, with your eyes focused on your feet, carefully raise your legs. Tuck your chin in slightly, straighten your back and slowly push your heels away from your body.

3 Hold the position for up to 5 breaths. Release gently out of the posture on the exhaling breath as you bend your knees and lower your feet.

1

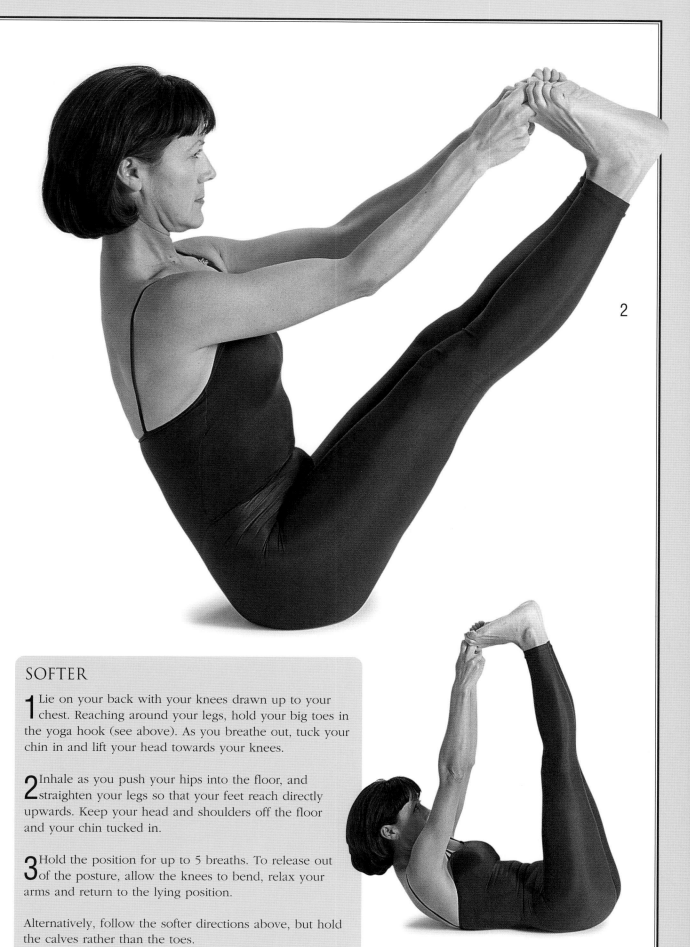

2

SOFTER

1 Lie on your back with your knees drawn up to your chest. Reaching around your legs, hold your big toes in the yoga hook (see above). As you breathe out, tuck your chin in and lift your head towards your knees.

2 Inhale as you push your hips into the floor, and straighten your legs so that your feet reach directly upwards. Keep your head and shoulders off the floor and your chin tucked in.

3 Hold the position for up to 5 breaths. To release out of the posture, allow the knees to bend, relax your arms and return to the lying position.

Alternatively, follow the softer directions above, but hold the calves rather than the toes.

CORPSE POSE II

SAVASANA

*The last posture of the sequence, we return to the corpse
pose which completely relaxes both the mind and the body.*

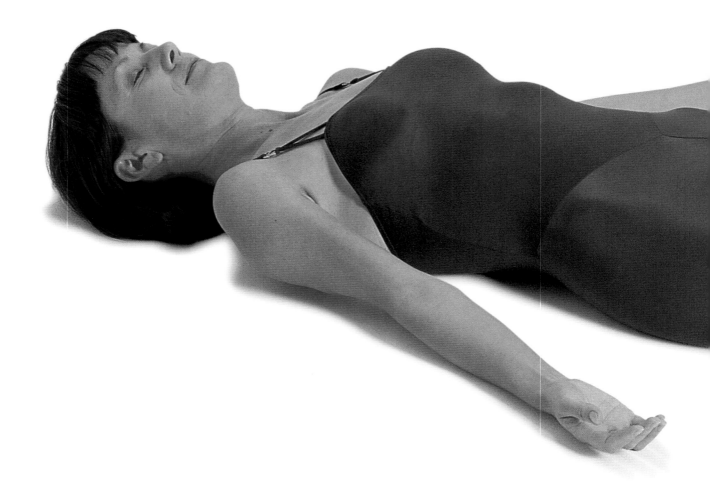

1 Lie on your back in the corpse pose, just as you
started this yoga practice. Your legs should be
relaxed with the feet falling outwards, your arms
by your sides with the hands relaxed and the
palms facing upwards. Let the fingers curl naturally.

2 Close your eyes, tuck your chin in a little,
spread your shoulders and lengthen your spine.

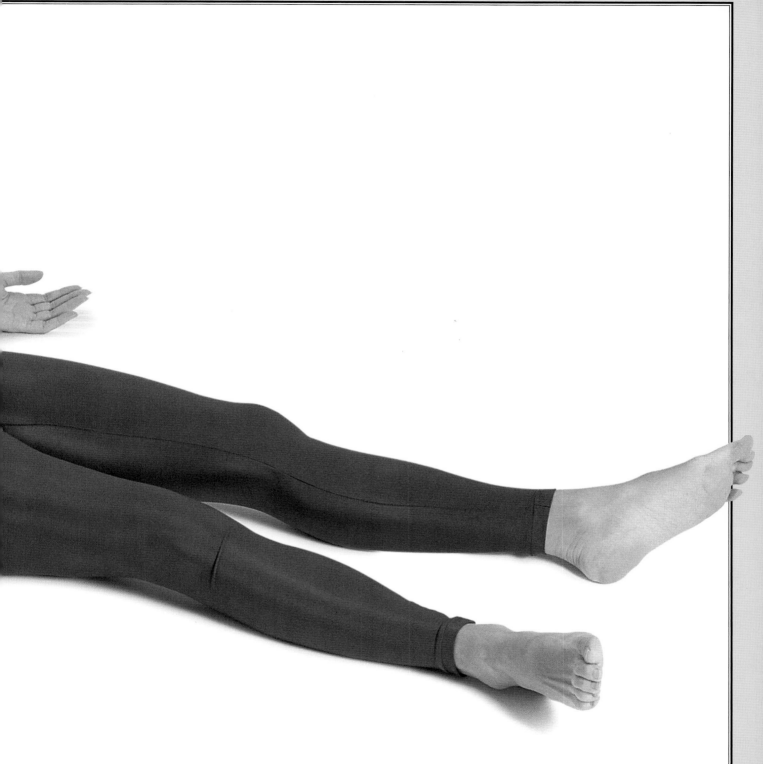

Now just let go ... surrender ... soften the face. Let the eyes, the brow and the ears melt back into the mat. Soften the jaw, unclench your teeth and let your tongue be soft in your mouth. Continue this softness down your throat and neck. Allow your shoulders to melt into the mat, relax your spine and soften your back muscles. Feel the lower back melt into the mat and let the hips open. Soften the buttocks, the abdomen and the thighs and let this softness continue down the legs, into the feet and the toes.

Completely surrender your body and let your thoughts float away like clouds. Allow yourself to relax completely for at least 5 minutes.

When you are ready, roll onto your right side and rest for a moment in this position as you bring your awareness back to the everyday world. Slowly come up to the sitting position and give yourself a few more moments, to feel completely at peace, positive about your life and your yoga practice.

SUN SALUTATION

SUYRA NAMASKAR

Begin by standing on your mat in Mountain Pose (Tadasana). Bring your feet together (toes and ankles touching) with your arms by your sides. Lengthen your spine upwards from the tip of the tailbone to the crown of the head. Inhale deeply.

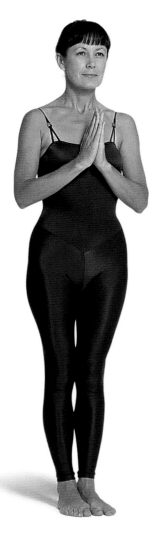

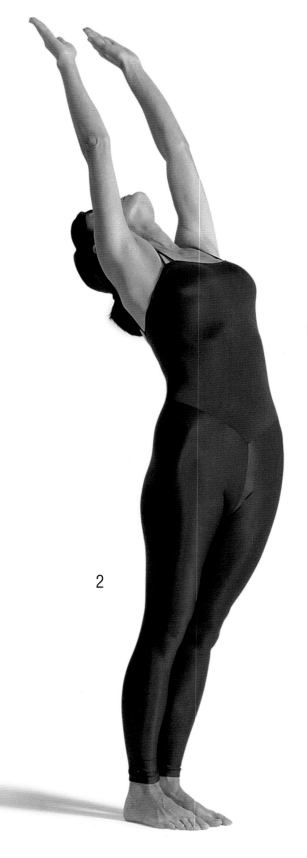

2

1 Exhale and bring the hands together in the 'prayer' position.

2 Inhale as you stretch your arms up beside your head, lengthening and arching your spine.

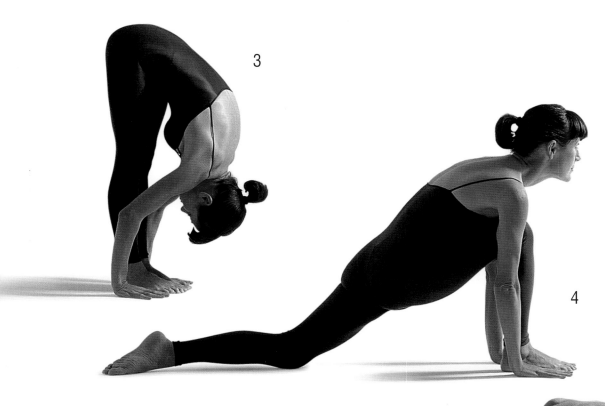

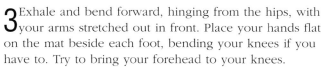

3 Exhale and bend forward, hinging from the hips, with your arms stretched out in front. Place your hands flat on the mat beside each foot, bending your knees if you have to. Try to bring your forehead to your knees.

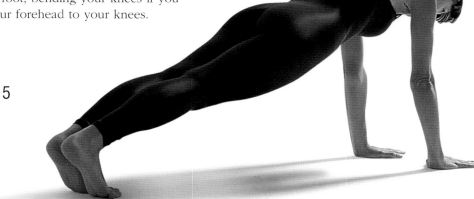

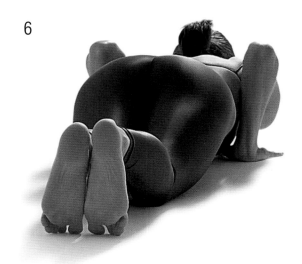

4 Inhale as you lunge back with the left foot as far as possible. Place your left knee on the mat, drawing the chest and the head upwards.

5 Hold your breath and bring both feet (with the toes tucked under) back into 'pole' position so that the body is in a straight line from head to heels, with your hands under your shoulders.

6 Maintaining the position of your hands and keeping your hips up, exhale as you bring your knees, chest and chin down to the mat.

SUN SALUTATION

(Continued)

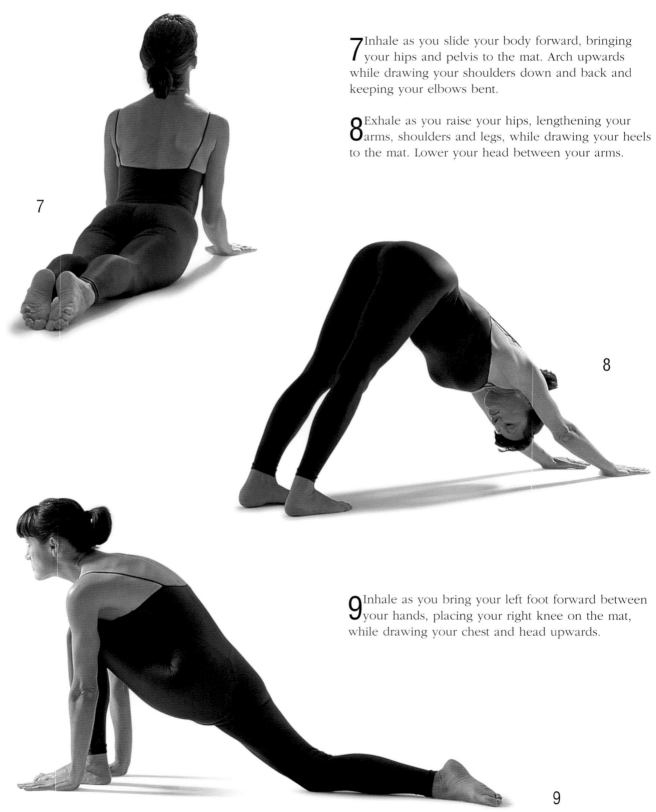

7 Inhale as you slide your body forward, bringing your hips and pelvis to the mat. Arch upwards while drawing your shoulders down and back and keeping your elbows bent.

8 Exhale as you raise your hips, lengthening your arms, shoulders and legs, while drawing your heels to the mat. Lower your head between your arms.

9 Inhale as you bring your left foot forward between your hands, placing your right knee on the mat, while drawing your chest and head upwards.

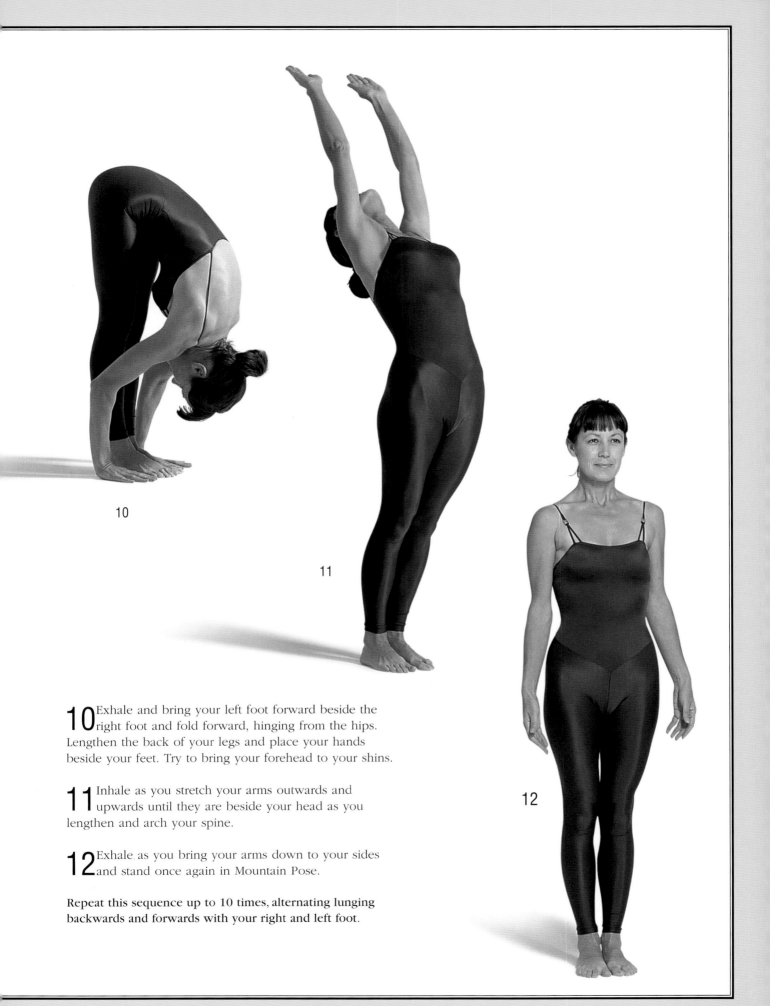

10
11
12

10 Exhale and bring your left foot forward beside the right foot and fold forward, hinging from the hips. Lengthen the back of your legs and place your hands beside your feet. Try to bring your forehead to your shins.

11 Inhale as you stretch your arms outwards and upwards until they are beside your head as you lengthen and arch your spine.

12 Exhale as you bring your arms down to your sides and stand once again in Mountain Pose.

Repeat this sequence up to 10 times, alternating lunging backwards and forwards with your right and left foot.

SALUTING THE SUN

COMPLETE SEQUENCE

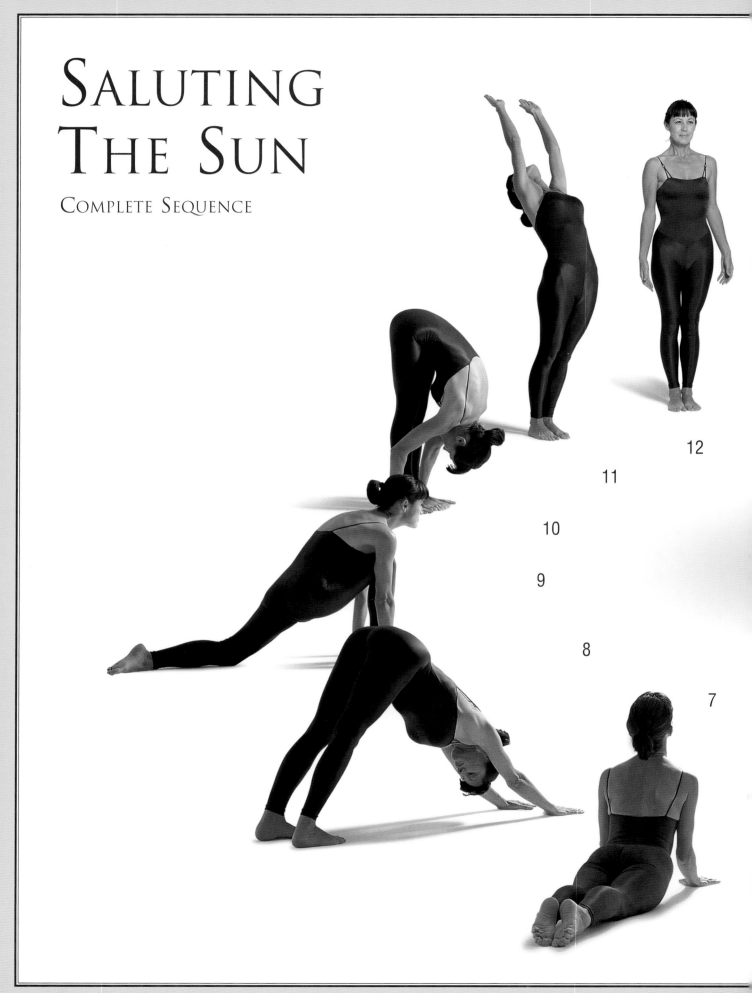

12

11

10

9

8

7

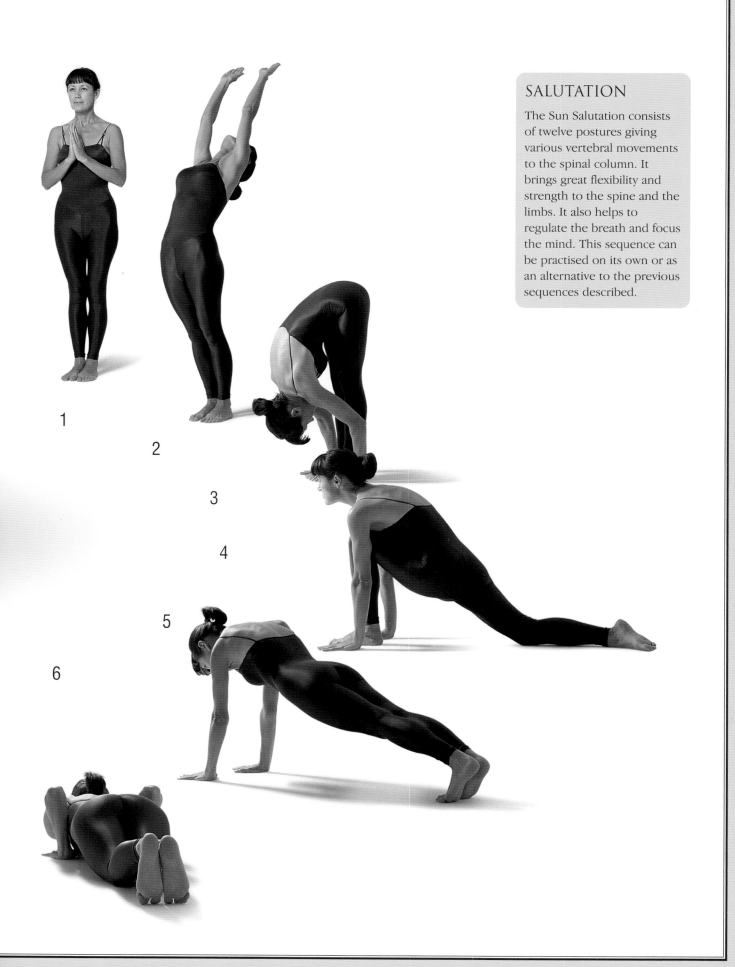

The Sun Salutation consists of twelve postures giving various vertebral movements to the spinal column. It brings great flexibility and strength to the spine and the limbs. It also helps to regulate the breath and focus the mind. This sequence can be practised on its own or as an alternative to the previous sequences described.

1

2

3

4

5

6

MEDITATION

CALMING THE MIND

A calming practice bringing increased mental clarity, increased energy levels and greater capacity for contentment.

The word meditation is naturally associated with the practice of Yoga. It describes a state of inner stillness, a feeling of balance and peace that, with regular practice, will radiate from one's daily routine into the everyday world of our busy lives. It is not the purpose of this book to explore meditation in any depth, but the following simple practice is one you might like to try while your body is feeling relaxed and alert at the end of the posture sequence. Or it can be practised on its own.

1 Make sure your surroundings are comfortably warm and quiet. Allow 5 to 10 minutes at first. Gradually increase the time to 20 minutes or more, as you feel able.

2 Sit comfortably with a straight back and with legs crossed. Rest the hands lightly on the knees or the thighs. Sitting on a firm pillow or a folded blanket can help you to keep your spine straight.

3 Close your eyes and gently bring your attention inward, away from the external world. Soften the face. Tuck your chin in. Relax your neck and shoulder muscles. Breathe gently and evenly.

4 Bring your awareness to any thoughts that come into your mind. See if you can simply observe them, letting them come, and letting them go, without following them. It's as if your mind is a beautiful, clear blue sky, and your thoughts are small, white clouds passing across it. Be patient with yourself. Your mind is used to getting its own way; some days your thoughts may be many and your mind might seem like an overcast sky. By quietly observing the thoughts they will slow down and become fewer. Enjoy the spaces between the thoughts. Allow that sense of peace and wellbeing to expand as your mind clears and becomes quiet.

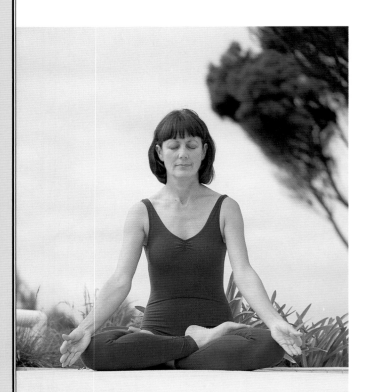

SOFTER

Sit on the floor against a wall with your back straight and legs either crossed or outstretched. Place a small cushion in the small of your back. OR – Sit on an upright chair with your back straight and your feet placed flat on the floor directly under your knees. Push your buttocks into the back of the chair. Use a folded blanket under the feet if your heels do not touch the floor.

A WORD ON DIET

Just as daily practice of the physical postures promotes health and wellbeing, a sensible diet enables the body to obtain maximum benefit from the food you eat. Your body needs food to be able to repair itself, and as fuel for energy. Simple, natural and wholesome foods that are easily digested will enhance your journey toward radiant physical health.

Rather than making a sudden decision to change your eating habits, which might not be easy to maintain, simply listen more closely to your body's needs, and alter your diet gradually when you feel ready. A gentle approach to change is often more practical and sustainable than a hasty one. If you are in any doubt, consult your health practitioner for guidance as to the right food requirements for your particular metabolism.

LASTLY ...

This book is a guide to yoga practice for those wishing to follow a routine at home. However there is no substitute for learning with a qualified yoga teacher. It is recommended that you take the time to find a teacher you can relate to and who teaches a style that is appropriate to your physical circumstances and also your temperament. You will discover that yoga teachers take many approaches. Some will focus more on

the mental aspects, some on the devotional path, and others on the physical forms of yoga. The sequence we have described is based on a gentle physical style of Hatha yoga. Check in your local directory to see what is available near you.

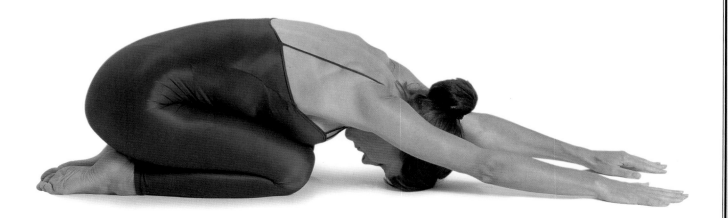

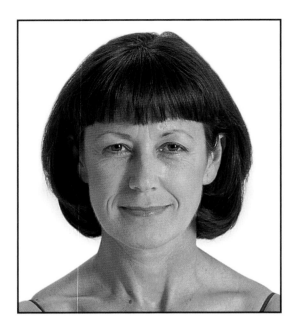

ABOUT THE AUTHOR

When Yolanda first discovered yoga she was in her mid-thirties. With no athletic or sporting background she could not even touch her toes. But she fell in love with yoga and took up formal studies both in Australia and in India. Now at 48, she teaches yoga from her studio in St Kilda, Melbourne. She hopes this book will encourage others to find good health, peace and harmony as she has, through yoga.

YOGA
CLASS

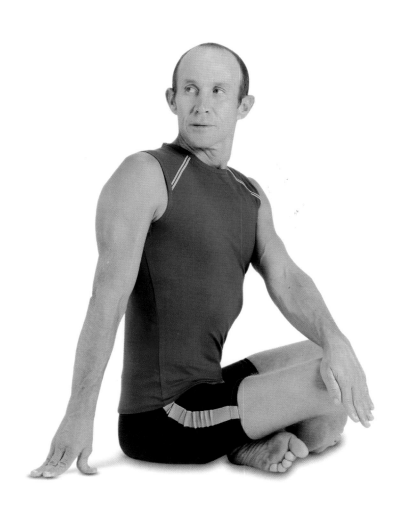

Art Director: Karen Moores
Graphic Artist: Post Pre-press Group
Photographer: UB Photo
Editor: Fiona Staun
Special thanks to Alida Hickey

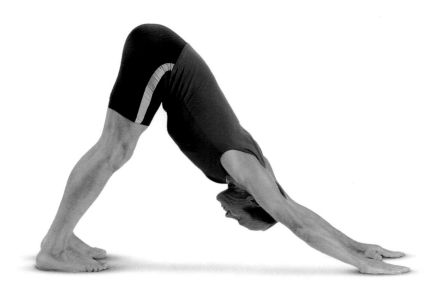

CONTENTS

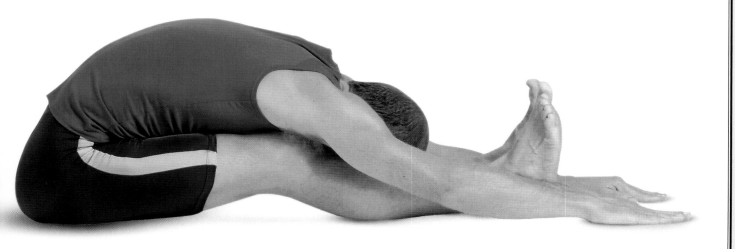

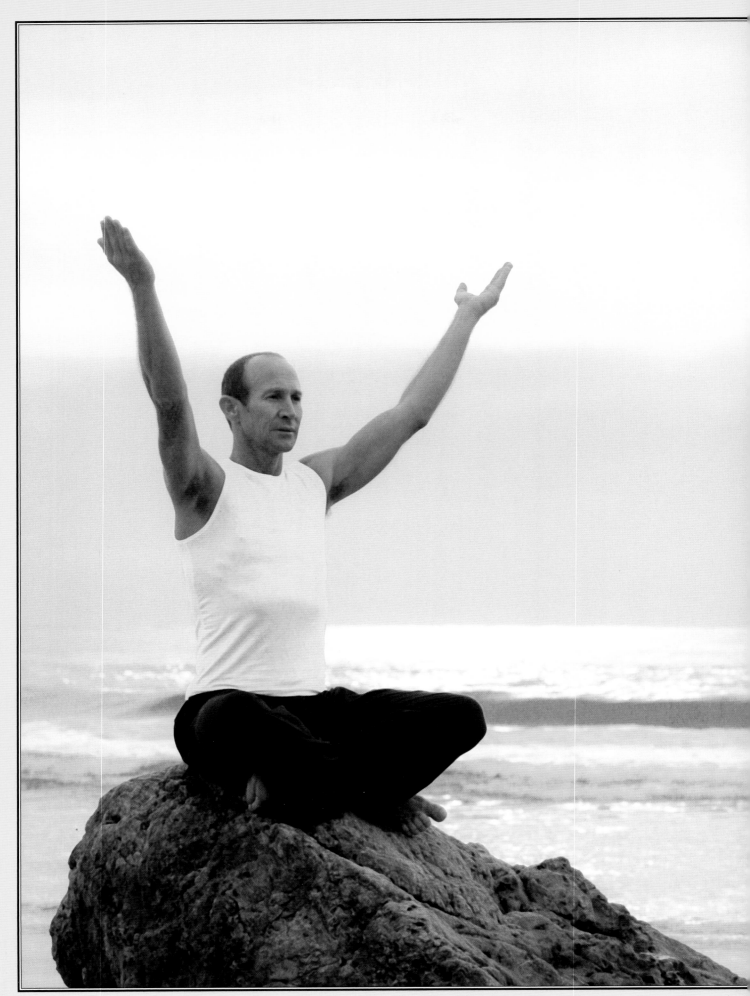

INTRODUCTION TO YOGA

Discover your journey to health and harmony

Yoga aims to bring a harmonious balance into our lives. It allows us to let go of the past and future, and to be in the present moment experiencing our true 'Inner Self'. Yoga starts us on the journey towards a healthy and harmonious life.

The word Yoga simply means *Union*. This union implies harmony of mind, body and spirit. It is not associated with any particular religion, or religious group. Yoga has been practiced and passed on for about 5000 years. Originating in India, the first references to yoga, its philosophy and its many postures were discovered in some of the oldest written manuscripts ever found.

YOGA CLASS

Yoga Class is a clear and comprehensive approach to yoga, incorporating some Chi Gung movements. You will find it designed for beginner and intermediate students. *Yoga Class* includes 'natural breathing' – a flowing series of postures and relaxation. It begins with a relaxation period, bringing awareness about our natural breath, followed by a gentle series of limbering up movements to open the joints, unblock and stimulate energy flow. It then moves through a flowing series of dynamic and static postures to cleanse and strengthen, whilst continuing to generate and circulate energy throughout the whole body. The sequence concludes with a meditation to centre the body and mind. Gary Bromley, a true Yoga expert, will gently guide you throughout.

People of all ages and walks of life can enjoy yoga. Don't be concerned if you are unable to perform some of the postures. *Yoga Class* is designed to allow you to work within your own boundaries and remain free from goals. Do not strain or force your body into a posture. With regular practice, your body will become stronger, more flexible, and energy will increase.

So begin your yoga journey with an open mind, allow change to happen and discover the wonderful joy yoga will bring to you.

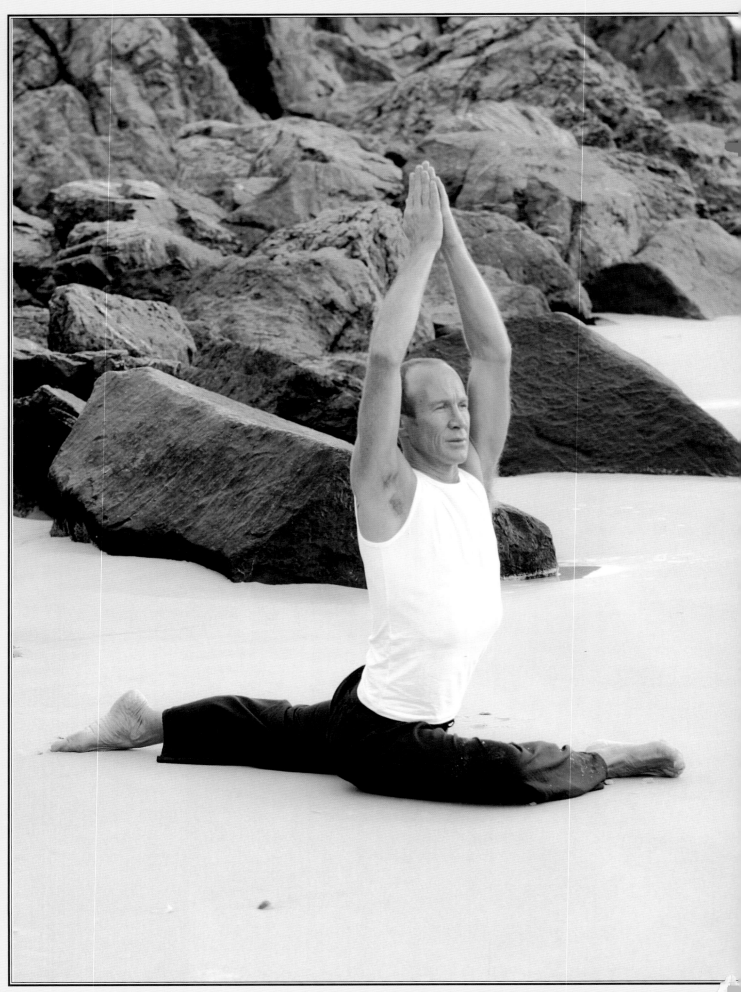

THE BENEFITS OF YOGA

Yoga helps us to balance our lives, to be happy and healthy and to improve our relationships with our partners, children, friends and ourselves.

YOGA LETS YOU REGAIN CONTROL

As yoga totally embraces our mind, body and spirit, you will find it helps improve relationships, sporting pursuits and our working lives.

Regular practice can help change a negative mindset by offering inner peace and an ability to face upheavals and deal with problems.

AN ABUNDANT LIFE

The benefits of Yoga seem to be endless. It is perfectly adaptable to all kinds of lifestyles – Eastern, Western, children and adults. It can replace the so-called buzzes of alcohol, caffeine, nicotine and other stimulants with a wonderful sense of invigoration. Sports people may find a new sense of energy release. It is a fabulous way to tone and strengthen our bodies.

WELLNESS – NOT ILLNESS

When you regularly practise yoga, you may find it:
- Helps relieve depression and anxiety
- Increases energy levels
- Aids weight control
- Helps relieve arthritis
- Boosts flexibility and energy
- Provides natural stimulation.
- Improves osteoporosis, circulation and digestion and lowers blood pressure

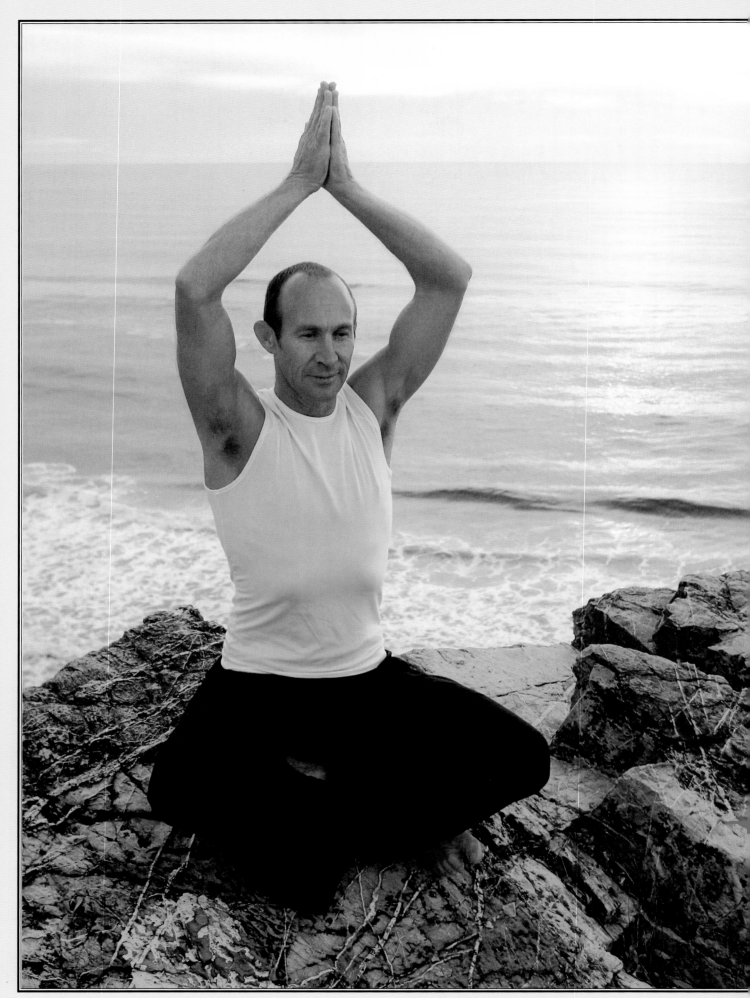

WHEN AND WHERE TO PRACTISE YOGA

Yoga is meant to be enjoyable, so it is important to approach your practice with a sense of adventure, purpose and respect.

A SPECIAL PLACE

Find yourself a really special place, as this is your 'time-out'. Make sure it is quiet and peaceful. You need to be comfortable. Rooms should be airy and dust-free. Place your mat towards a door or window. If outside, make sure the conditions are pleasant and face away from the sun, preferably towards a tree or water.

A SPECIAL TIME

Ideal times for yoga are early morning or early evening.

A SPECIAL WAY

Yoga is best practised on an empty stomach. In the morning, just have a glass of warm water with lemon on rising. It is best to wait three or four hours after a meal, but some practices can be done after a 'light' meal. A 'bathroom' stop is recommended before you start, too.

A SPECIAL OUTFIT

It is important to wear loose, comfortable clothing when doing yoga. You don't need to buy special clothing, but remember there is lots of sitting, standing and stretching. Take off any jewellery and metal items, and tie the hair back loosely. You also need to stay warm after your session.

WHAT YOU NEED

All you need for the yoga experience is a towel, mat, pillow and a chair – things so easily available.

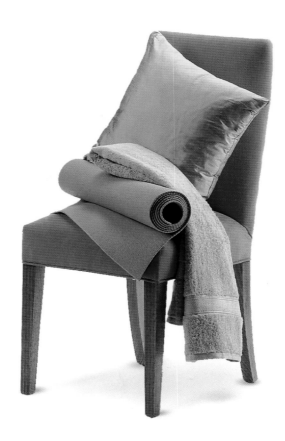

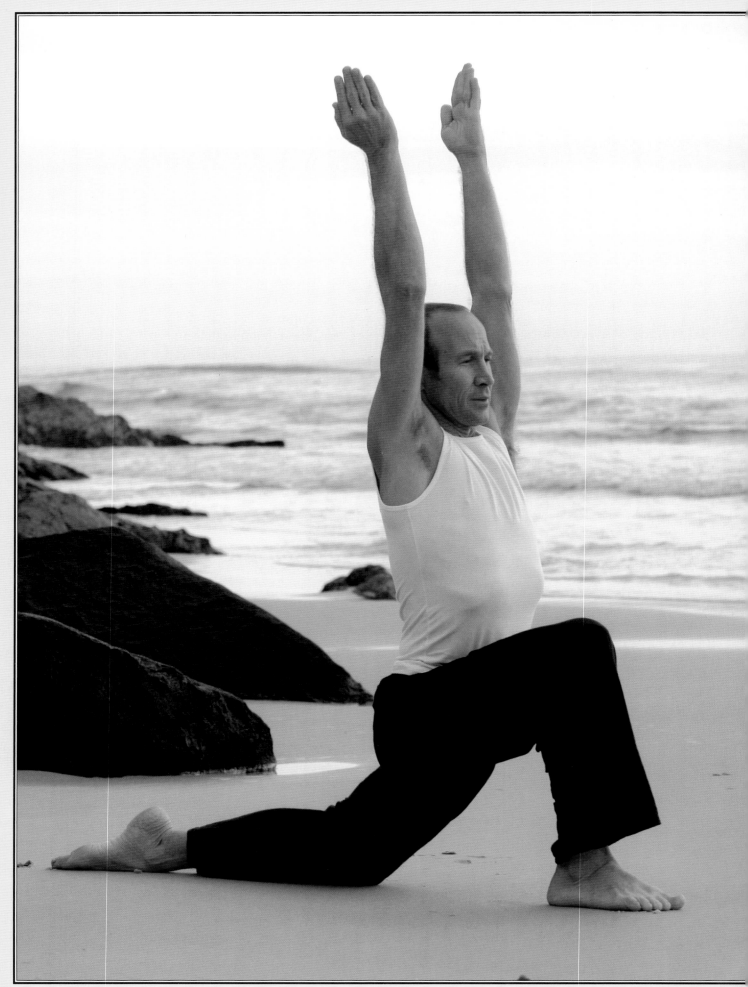

THE NATURAL BREATH

From the moment of birth, we take our first breath, filling our body with life force. As we continue our life journey, not a minute of the day passes, without us giving nourishment to our body and mind via the breath. Unfortunately, that quality of nourishment can diminish, as we get caught up in the cobweb of life. Our fast pace of life tends to place increasing stress on our bodies, directly and indirectly affecting many physiological processes.

EFFECTS OF STRESS

One of the first reactions to stress in the body is the over-stimulation of our sympathetic nervous system. The diaphragm begins to constrict and sets up rapid shallow breathing. Unbelievably, a vast range of illnesses can occur from this simple reaction. Other factors such as poor posture, diet, muscle tone and emotional responses, can all have an effect on the way we breathe.

BREATH OF LIFE

Being able to breathe correctly will make an enormous difference to your overall health and emotional state. First, breathe in through the nose. Feel the breath below the abdomen. The abdomen will rise on inhalation, then feel the lungs expand like a balloon. When you exhale (through the nose), release your chest and abdomen. Remember not to control or force the breath. Simply observe and feel its rhythmic inhalation and exhalation.

BREATH FOR YOGA

Use your breath as a valuable tool during your Yoga practice. Feel areas of tightness, tension or resistance release with each breath. Experience the flow of energy throughout the body. Avoid trying to force your body deeper into postures which can create further resistance. Learn to use the breath as a tool to create support for your movements, and to release the whole body. Breathing 'naturally' will allow you to experience a more balanced life. It will help you release tension and stress, allow your whole body to function more effectively and clear your mind.

PEACEFUL POSE

SHAVASANA

Relaxes the whole body and mind. Ideally practised before a session to let go of all tension and to bring awareness onto the natural flow of breath below the navel.

1 Lie flat on your back, with legs straight and hip width apart. Allow your legs and feet to roll away from each other, with your arms alongside your body, palms up at a 30–45 degree angle.

2 Gently elongate your neck and tuck your chin in slightly. Close your eyes, feel your posterior body sinking into the floor, and your anterior light and weightless.

3 Bring your awareness onto your natural flow of breath below your navel. Do not try to force or control your breath. Allow your mind to follow the rhythm of your breath and experience the present moment. A state of stillness, peace and inner harmony.

4 Place your right hand below your navel, palm down and left on top. Continue to observe the rising of your abdomen on the inhale and the falling on exhale. Continue for 3–5 minutes before opening your eyes, bending your knees and rolling to your right side coming up to Mountain Pose.

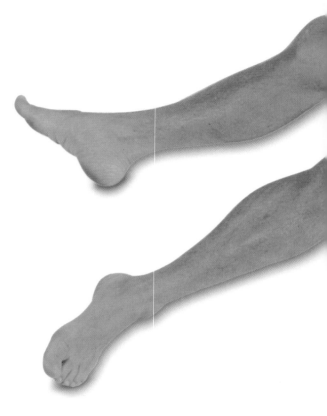

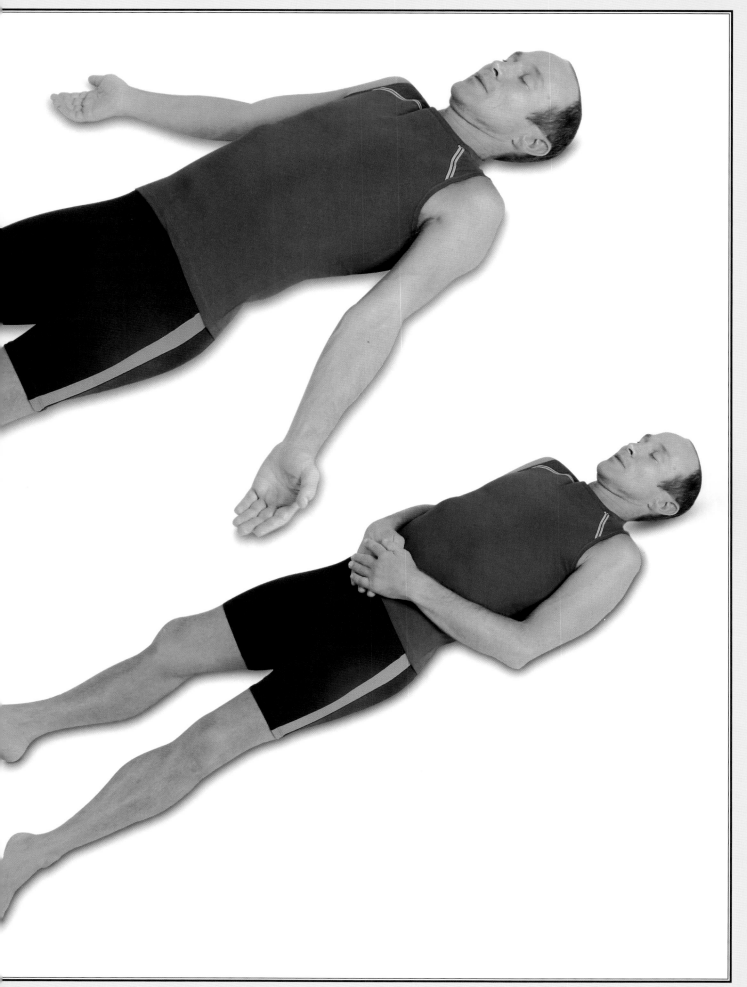

MOUNTAIN POSE

WITH HANDS IN PRAYER POSE

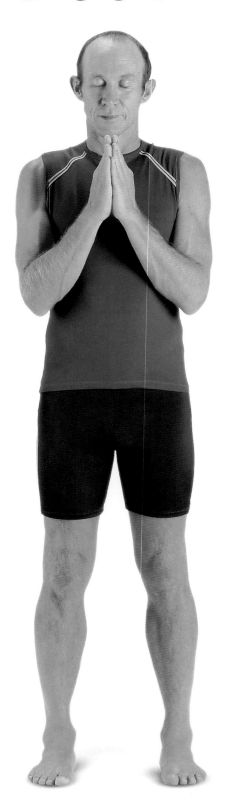

Benefits:

• Bringing your hands into Prayer Pose allows
  your body/mind to centre
• Harmonises your nervous system
• Energises your heart, pericardium and lungs

1 Stand in Mountain Pose (Page 79) with hands in
Prayer Pose. Relax shoulders and lengthen your spine.

2 Close your eyes and continue to observe your natural
breath flow. Remain for 30 seconds.

MOUNTAIN POSE

TADASANA

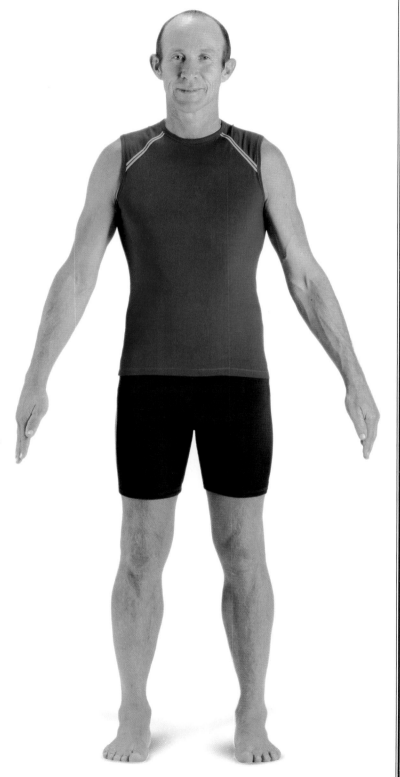

Benefits:
- Tadasana is used as a foundation of all the standing postures and movements
- The natural way to stand – 'a relaxed and steady standing position'
- Cultivates a sense of strength and stability
- Mountain Pose is an effective way of freeing energy that has been blocked by stress and tension
- The primary posture for the absorption of universal energy

1 Begin with your feet between your hips and shoulders – go with what feels natural and comfortable. Slightly angle your feet outwards with your weight evenly spread through the balls, lateral edge and heel. Avoid your arches collapsing inwards. Try to feel them lift up.

2 Unlock your knee joints and tuck your sacrum slightly in. Relax your abdomen and hips.

3 Lengthen up through the spine. Let your arms hang and relax your shoulders.

4 Slightly tuck your chin in, and at the same time, feel the back of your neck lengthen.

5 Soften your eyes, face and relax your jaw. Gaze forward and downward. You should feel as if your head is being suspended from above, at the crown, by an invisible string.

6 Feel energy permeating your body, through the pores of your skin – producing a light, free feeling. Remain for 3 to 5 minutes. Your eyes can remain open or closed.

LIMBERING UP EXERCISES

PAWANMUKTASANA SERIES

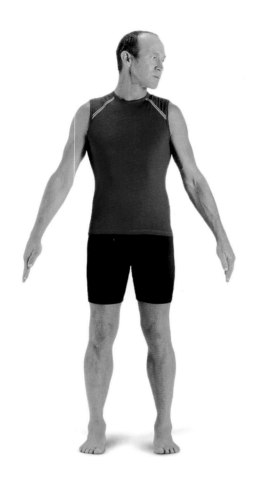 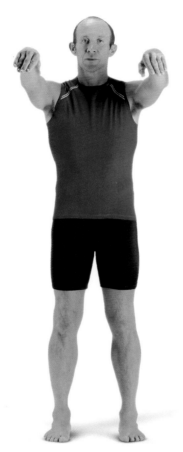 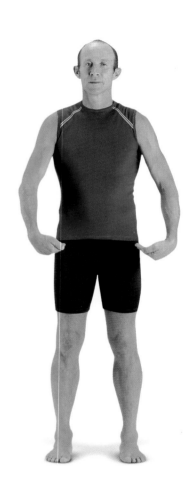

1 Begin in Mountain Pose (Page 79). Lower your chin down to your chest and roll your head in a circular pathway to the right. Elongate your neck as it passes the centre position. Repeat 3 times and alternate to the left. Be careful not to bend your neck backwards.

2 Float your arms up to shoulder height, palms down. Swing them behind and out to the side of your body. Repeat 5 times. Roll your shoulders backwards 5 times, alternating shoulders 5 times.

3 Rotate your wrist joint 5 times and alternate. Open and close your hands, stretch through the fingers. Shake your hands to shoulder height and back alongside the body. Relax your face and body.

Benefits:
- Opens your joints and makes your muscles and connective tissue supple
- Stimulates the flow of blood, lymph and cerebrospinal fluid
- Unblocks and stimulates the flow of energy through the meridians
- Warming up helps prepare your body to avoid injury

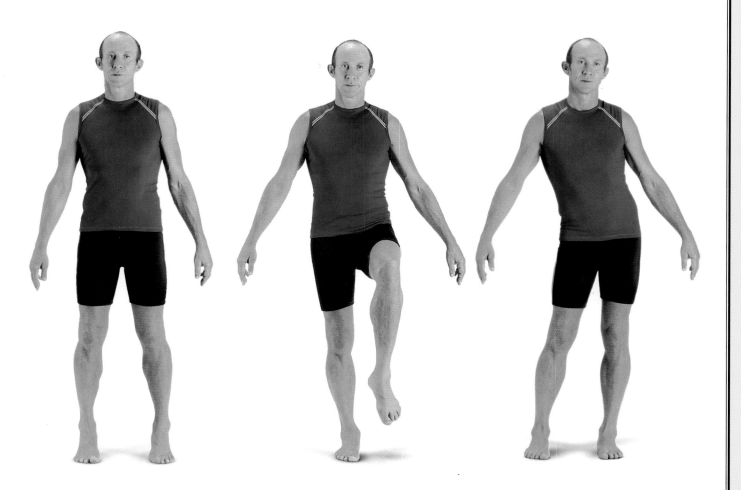

4 Rise onto the balls of your feet, keep your weight even behind the big and little toe. Lower back onto your heels and sink slightly bending your knees. Take care to keep your knees over and behind your toes as you sink. Repeat 5 times.

5 Raise your left leg in front of your body; flex and extend your ankle joint, and then rotate your foot in a circle. Repeat with the right ankle.

6 From Mountain Pose move your hips in a small circle clockwise. Do 5 times clockwise and alternate.

LIMBERING UP EXERCISES

(continued)

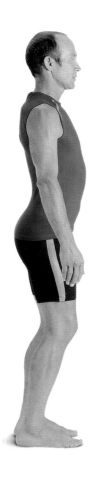 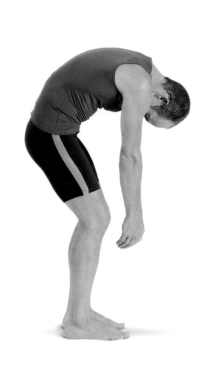 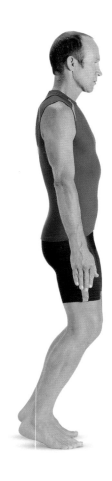

7 Using small movements, tuck your pelvis back and under. Keep your upper body stationary. Repeat 5 times. Extend the front of your chest forward, and then lower your chin into your chest. Relax your shoulders. Repeat 5 times.

8 Bend your knees, lower your chin into your chest, relax your shoulders and vertebra-by-vertebra roll down. Keep your knees bent, push through your feet and reverse the downward path back to Mountain Pose. Repeat 3 times.

9 From Mountain Pose, rock forward onto your toes and back onto your heels. Keep the spine lengthened.

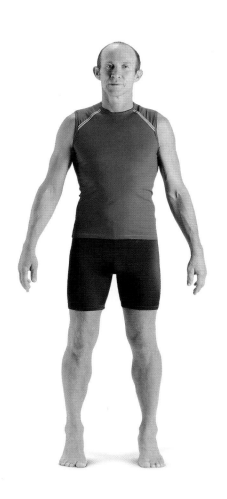

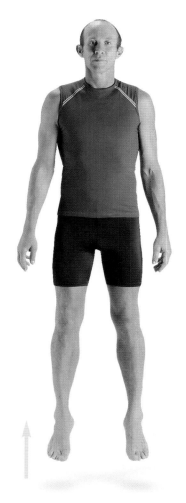

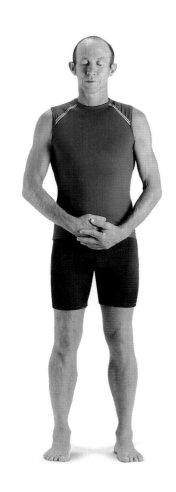

10 Keep your feet grounded and move your body in a bouncing action. Have awareness of fascia releasing. Continue bouncing on the balls of your feet. Keep them grounded, whilst keeping your heels off the ground.

11 From bouncing, continue into small jumps. Keep your ankle and knee joints soft.

SOFTER
Stop at step 10 if you have discomfort.

12 Stand in Mountain Pose, place your right hand below the navel and left hand on top. 'Gather the Chi' and allow your diaphragm to come back to its natural rhythm. Hold for 60 seconds and roll down to Diamond Pose.

DIAMOND POSE

VAJRASANA

Benefits

- Improves flexibility of your spine, ankles, knees, and hips
- Assists digestion and assimilation, both psychological and physiologically
- A meditative pose
- Opens and circulates energy – main central energy channel
- Strengthens and tones your abdomen and spine

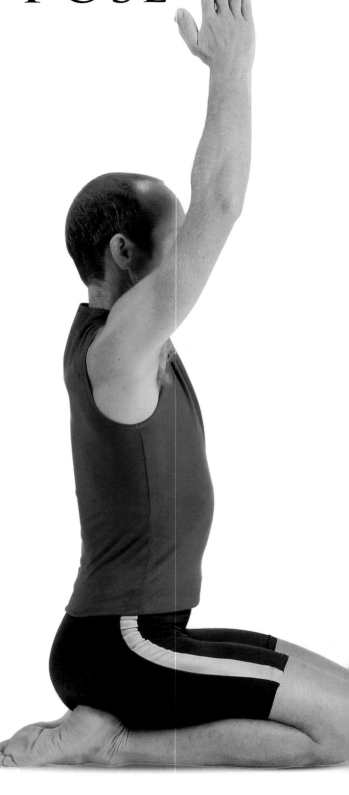

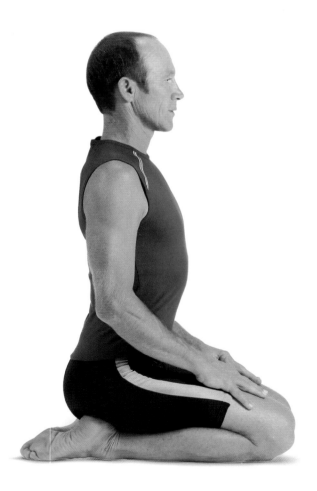

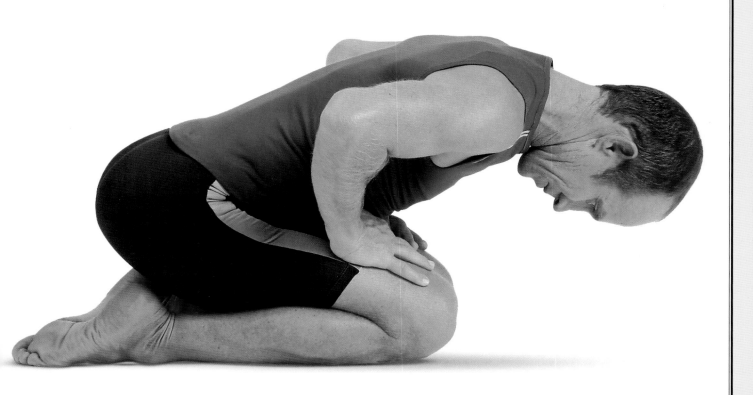

STATIC VERSION

1 Kneel on the floor, with your knees and ankles slightly apart. Rest your buttocks on your heels and your palms down on your thighs.

2 Feel your spine and neck lengthening with your chin slightly tucked. Relax your shoulders.

DYNAMIC VERSION

1 Start in Diamond Pose, and then extend your arms overhead bringing your palms together and taking them down through your torso.

2 Rest your palms on your thighs and fold forward from your hips. Keep lengthening through your spine until your lower back releases. Then tuck your chin into your chest and roll up. Repeat 3 to 5 times in a flowing manner.

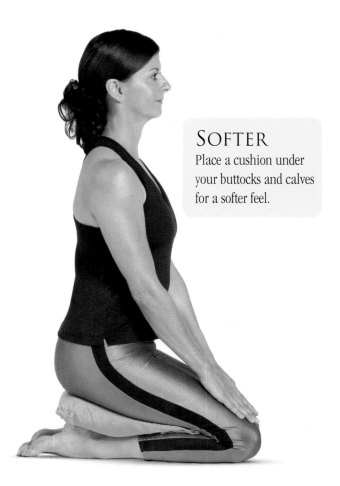

SOFTER
Place a cushion under your buttocks and calves for a softer feel.

CAT POSE

BIDALASANA

Benefits
- Gentle movement through your spine, shoulders and hips
- Improves blood flow to your spine and spinal nerves
- Strengthens, tones and stretches your abdominal organs and spine
- Improves spinal flexibility
- Opens up your bladder and stomach meridians

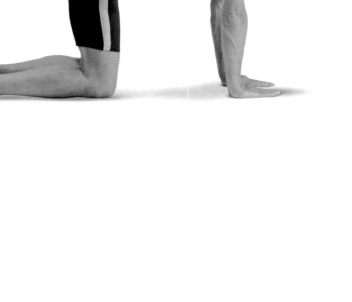

DYNAMIC VERSION

1 Start on all fours with knees under hips and hands under shoulders. Make sure your head, neck and spine are parallel to the ground.

2 Take your navel towards the ground and lift your tailbone– feel your sitting bones spread. Avoid taking your head back and continue to lengthen through your crown.

3 Tuck your chin in and round your spine. Feel your navel being drawn up and your buttocks contracting. Repeat, alternating the hollowing and rounding of your spine, five times.

STATIC VERSION

1 Hold Dynamic (step 2) for 10 seconds.

2 Then Dynamic (step 3) for 10 seconds and fold back into Hare Pose. (Page 88)

Avoid any tension while holding the poses.

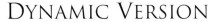

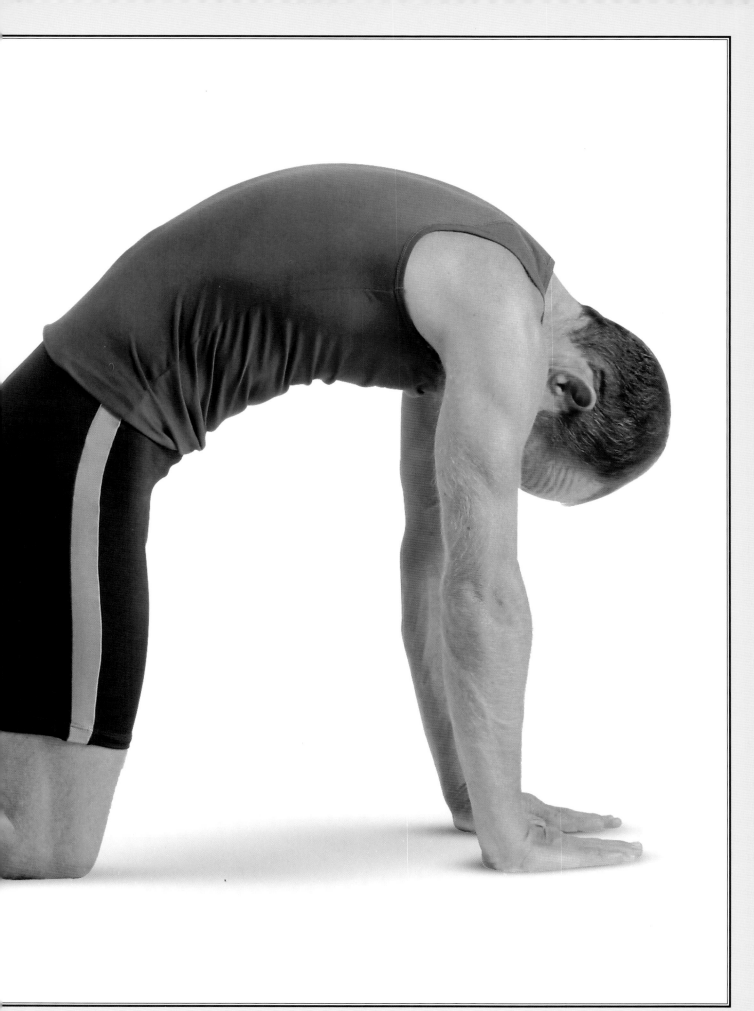

HARE POSE

SHASHANKASANA

Benefits
- Stretches your lower back
- Relaxes your sciatic nerves
- Strengthens and cleanses your lower lungs
  and stomach
- Opens the main central energy

1 From Cat Pose (Page 86, step 3) take your buttocks back to your heels. Keep your spine rounded, chin tucked into your chest and keep your hands stationary.

2 Keep your abdomen off your thighs. Hold for 10 seconds.

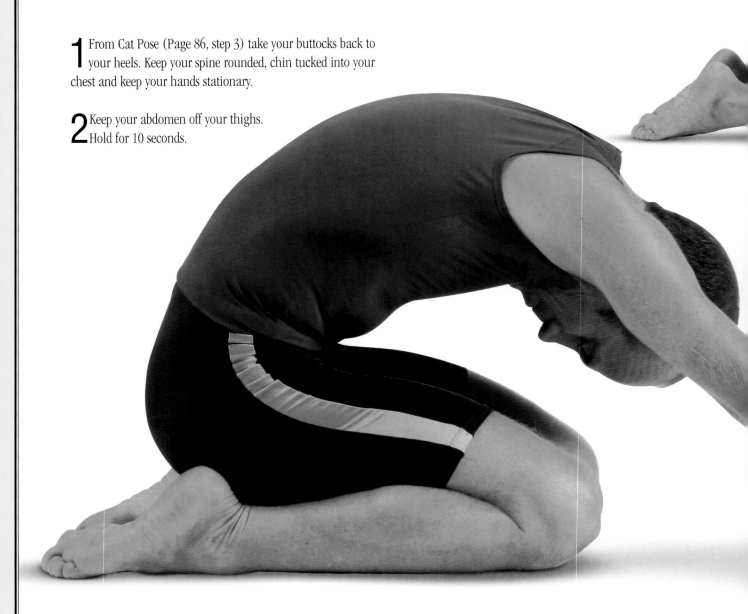

LIZARD POSE

UTTHAN PRISHASANA

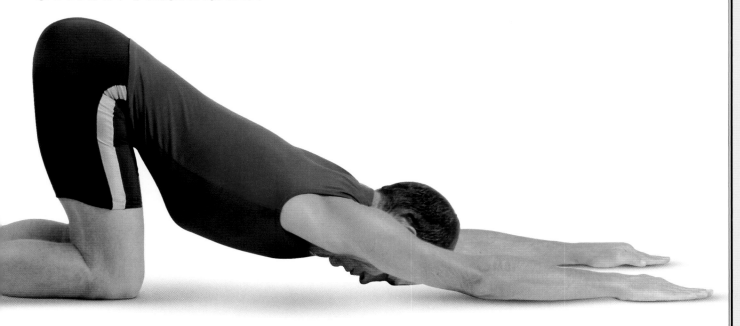

Benefits
- Exercises and strengthens your lungs and tones your entire back, especially your nerves and muscles
- Can relieve backache and fatigue
- Cleanses your lungs, liver, spleen and stomach

1 Slide your arms forward from Hare Pose until your thighs remain at right angles to the ground.

2 Rest your forehead on the ground and feel the front of your upper chest release towards the ground.

3 Relax your shoulders and hold for 10 seconds.

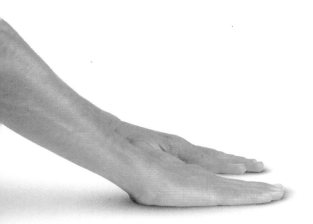

CHILD'S POSE

SUPTA VAJRASANA

Benefits
- A relaxation pose that has a calming effect on your nervous system
- Gently opens your hips and entire spine
- Strengthens your kidneys

1 Take your buttocks back to your heels, placing your forehead on the ground. Rest your hands palms down alongside your face.

2 Relax your shoulders and allow your whole body to soften. Hold for 20 seconds.

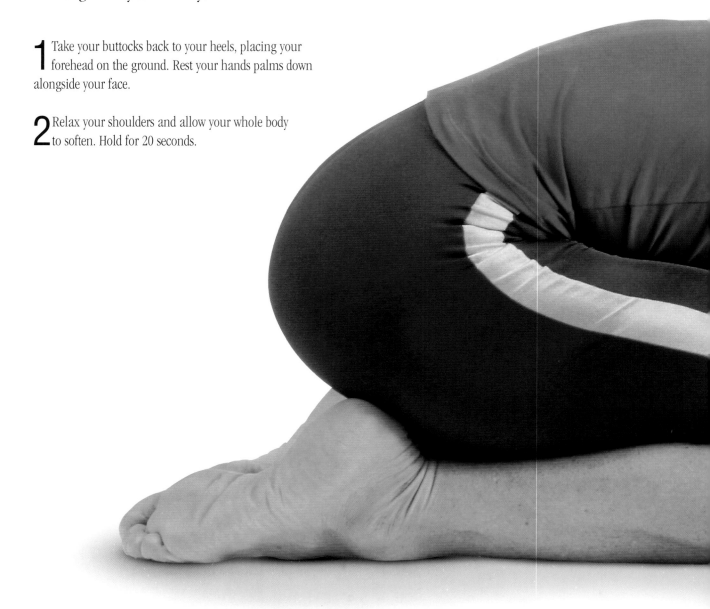

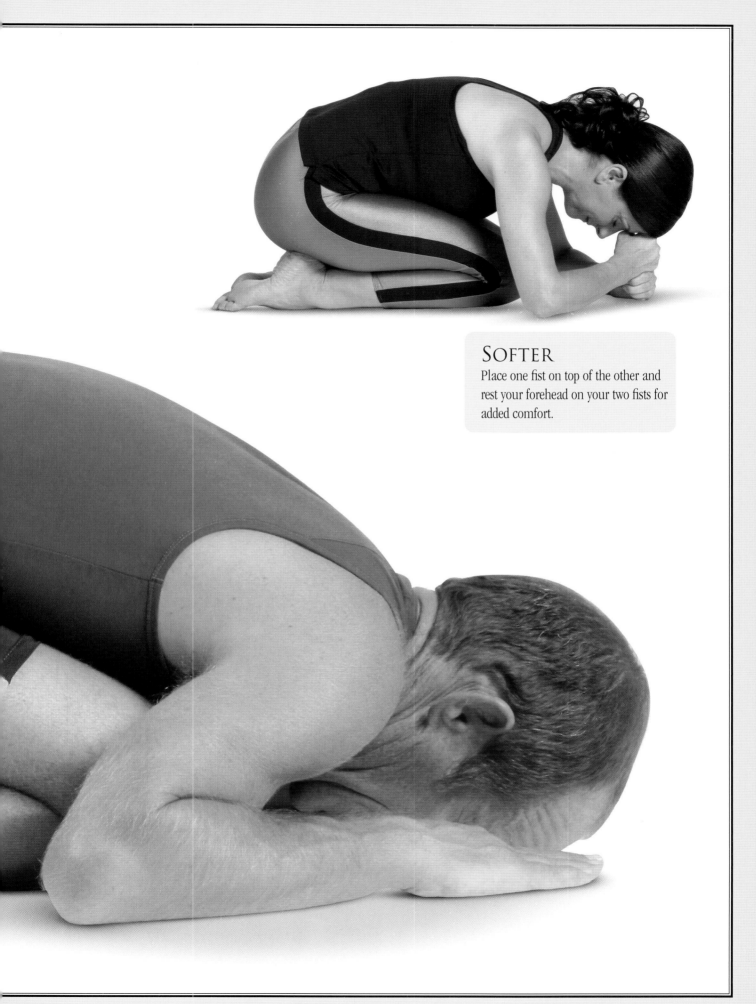

SOFTER
Place one fist on top of the other and rest your forehead on your two fists for added comfort.

EAGLE FOLDING ITS WINGS

Benefits

- Strengthens and tones your spine, buttocks and abdominal muscles
- Improves flexibility through your spine and back of your legs
- Opens up the flow of energy in all your meridians and vessels
- Increases circulation throughout your body
- Stimulates your endocrine system

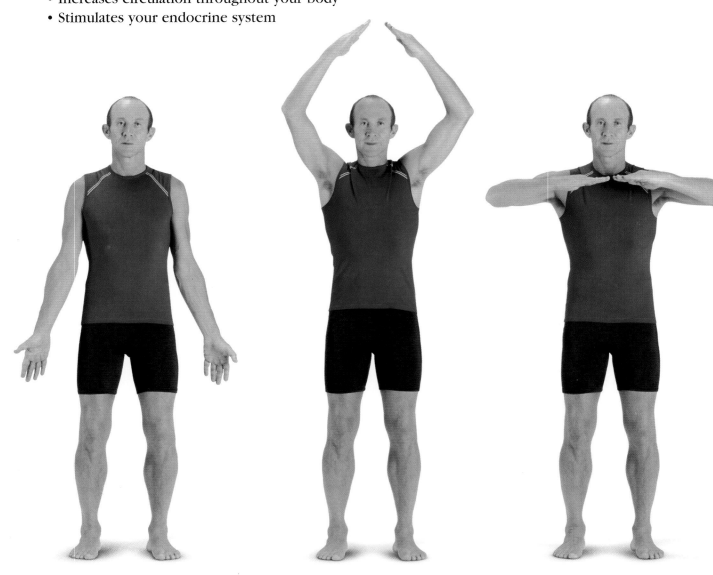

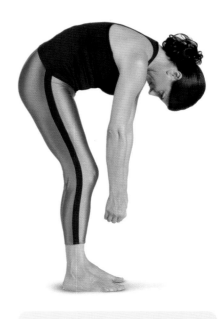

1 Begin in Mountain Pose (Page 79). Sink slightly, turn your palms out and raise your arms above your head, rising with the arm movement. Sink as you bring your arms down in front of your torso, palms down. Place the back of your hands in the small of your back. Check that your knees are behind and aligned with your toes.

2 Keeping your head, neck and back vertical, fold forward from the hip joint with a Monkey Back (Page 96, step 2). When your torso is at a right angle to the ground, continue the downward motion by tucking your chin in. Feel your lower back release and roll your shoulders, allowing your arms to come forward under your shoulders palms up.

3 With the knees bent and weight evenly under your feet, keep your chin tucked in and roll up to Mountain Pose. Repeat 3 times.

SOFTER

If you experience pain or tightness at step 2 leave your arms to the side, tuck your chin in and roll down. Continue step 3.

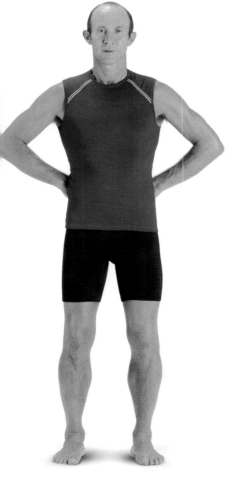

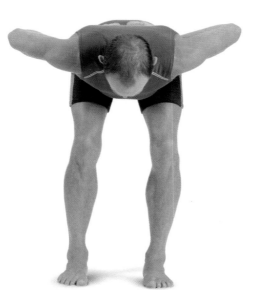

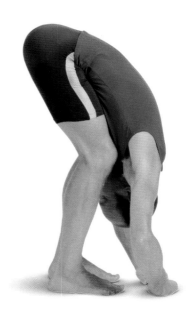

TORTOISE SERIES

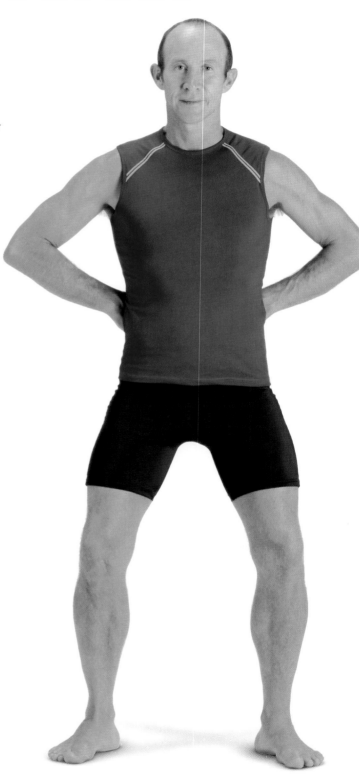

Benefits

- Strengthens and tones your spine, abdomen and legs
- Stretches your spine and back of your legs
- Circulates blood and energy around your body
- Strengthens your kidneys, lungs and heart
- Opens your kidney, liver, spleen and bladder meridians

1 Begin in Mountain Pose and turn your left foot out approximately half a hip width. Turn your feet to be on a 30 to 45 degree angle. Sink down slightly, bending your knees and keeping your weight evenly distributed under your feet. Place the back of your hands in the small of your back.

2 Keeping your body vertical, fold from your hip joint until at a right angle to the ground (The Tortoise). Look to the ground between your legs and feel your spine lengthen. Keep the natural lumber curve in your spine and check your knees are behind and aligned with your toes. Hold for 10 seconds.

3 Tucking your chin into your chest, fold forwards rolling your shoulders and bringing your hands (palms up) to relax on the ground. Keep your knees bent and feel the stretch through your spine (Tortoise Forward Bend). Hold for 10 to 20 seconds.

4 From the Tortoise Forward Bend, slowly sink your buttocks towards the ground to an approximate 45 degree angle and return to the starting position. Repeat 5 times slowly and hold the fifth squat (Tortoise Squat). Check your knee-toe alignment. Hold for 5 seconds.

5 From the Tortoise Squat, return to a Tortoise Forward Bend and lengthen through your legs and spine. Keep your knee joints unlocked. Hold for 10 to 20 seconds and roll back up to starting position.

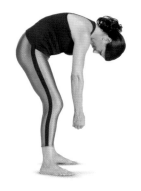
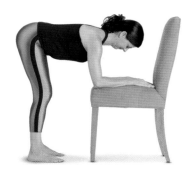

SOFTER

If your hips and spine are tight, leave out step 2 and roll down, continue step 3. Another option until your spine and hips gain strength and suppleness is to use a chair. If step 4 creates strain leave it out of your practice, until you are ready.

CAUTION

If you suffer from any condition where your head should not be below the level of your heart, bend half way only.

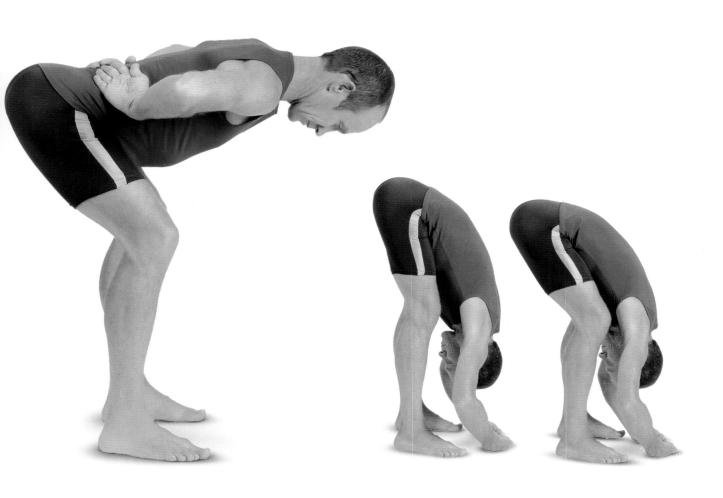

MONKEY SERIES

Benefits
- Has all the benefits of the Tortoise series (Page 94)
- Gives a gentle massage to your liver and spleen, and aids digestion
- Has a calming influence on your nervous system.
- Helps with anxiety and depression

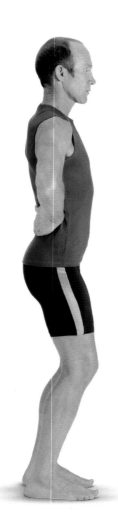

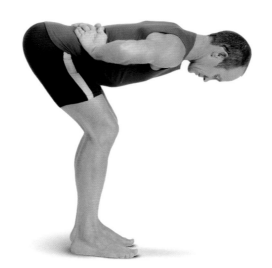

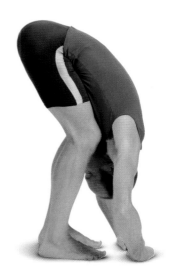

1 Begin in Mountain Pose, sink down slightly, bending your knees and keeping your weight evenly distributed under your feet. Place your hands in the small of your back.

2 Keep your spine vertical and fold forward from your hips. When your torso is at a right angle to the ground, hold statically (The Monkey). Check your knees are over and behind your toes. Hold for 10 seconds.

3 Release your lower back, tuck your chin in and roll forward. Place your hands (palms up) on the ground (Monkey Forward Bend). Keeping your torso centered between your legs, extend through the back of your legs. Check your knee joints are soft and unlocked. Hold for 10 seconds.

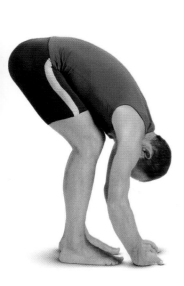

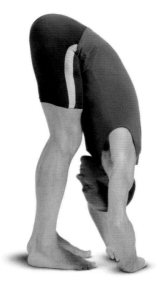

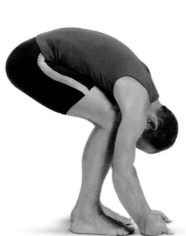

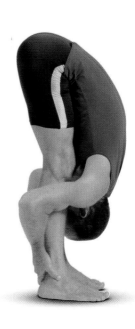

4 Bend your knees a little more and concentrate on stretching your sacrum and lower back. Hold for 10 seconds.

5 Maintaining the stretch on your lower back, slowly begin to lengthen the backs of your legs. You should feel an equal stretch on both. Hold for 10 seconds.

6 From Monkey Forward Bend, slowly lower your buttocks 90° to the ground, and in a continuous movement, rise back to starting position. Repeat 5 times and hold the fifth squat for 5 seconds. Check your knee alignment and keep your weight even under your feet.

7 From the Monkey Squat, place your hands around the outside of your ankles and lengthen through the back of the legs, into a Monkey Forward Bend. Relax your neck and shoulders and feel the crown of your head release towards the ground. Keep your knee joints unlocked. Hold for 10 seconds. Bend your knees, repeat step 4 and roll back up to Mountain Pose.

PALM TREE

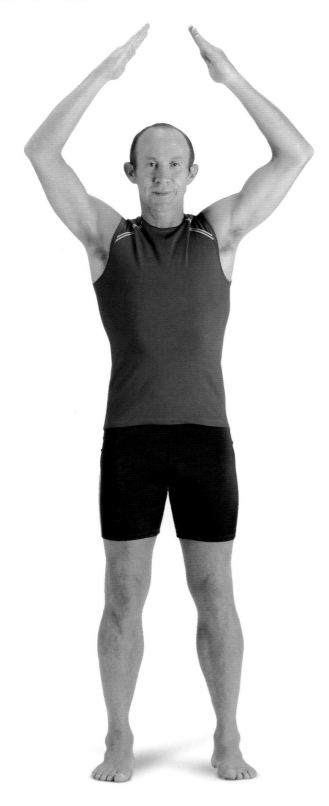

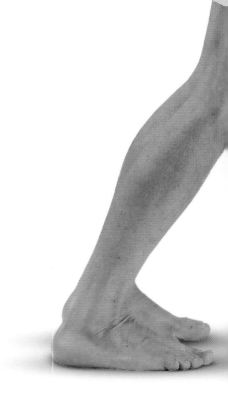

Benefits
- Counter posture for forward bends
- Lengthens your spine
- Strengthens your upper body
- Promotes better body alignment and the even muscle development on both sides of your body
- Opens and strengthens your heart and lungs

1 Roll up from Monkey Forward Bend – raise your arms overhead with your elbows bent and palms facing inwards.

2 Keep your sacrum slightly tucked and feel the lengthening through your spine.

DOWNWARD DOG

ADHO MUKHA SVANANA

Benefits

- Stretches your Achilles' tendons, hamstring and calf muscles. Tones your sciatic nerve
- Strengthens your upper body. Stretches and relaxes your spine
- Improves your circulation to your brain
- Opens your bladder, gallbladder, heart and lung meridian

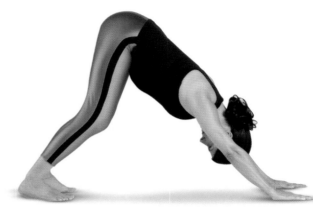

SOFTER

If you have tight hamstrings or hip flexors, keep your knees very bent.

CAUTION

Avoid if you have high blood pressure or a heart condition.

1 Roll down onto all fours. Tuck your toes under and push back with your hands while raising your hips up and back.

2 Press your heels towards the ground, keeping your knees slightly bent. Aim to distribute your weight evenly between hands and feet, so that your body forms an inverted 'V'.

3 Relax your neck muscles and roll your shoulders inwards, spreading your shoulder blades. Hold for 10 seconds.

THE CRESCENT MOON

CHANDRASANA

Benefits
- Stretches and opens your hips and helps relieve sciatica
- Increases the circulation to your pelvic area
- Strengthens your digestive system, heart, liver and lungs
- Helps improve concentration and balance to the nervous system

1 From Downward Dog, kneel on all fours or in a flowing action, bring your left leg forward. Point your toes on the right foot behind you. Your left knee is placed directly over your heel, feel the front of your right hip release. Your hands and fingers are placed on either side of your left foot, with fingers pointing forward.

2 When you are stable, bring your torso into an upright position and place your left hand on your thigh, right hand on top. Keep your pelvis stable and lengthen up through the spine. Eyes looking forward. Hold for 10 seconds.

3 Keep lifting your chest up as you extend your arms up, lengthening from your shoulders. Relax your shoulders away from the ears and keep the stretch through your spine. Hold for 10 seconds.

4 Bring your arms down and place your hands under your shoulders (fingers forward). Move your left leg back and come into Downward Dog (Page 99). Hold for 5 seconds and repeat steps 1 to 4 using your right leg.

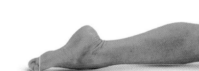

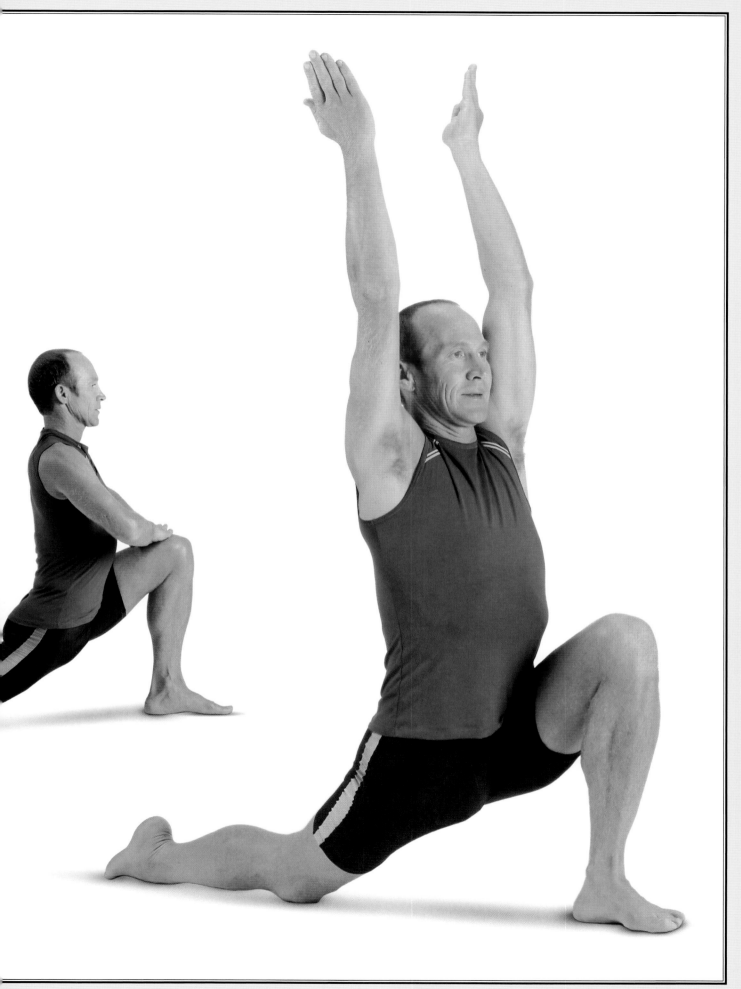

VINE POSE

GARUDASANA

Benefits
- Stretches your ankles, knees and hips
- Strengthens and opens your thoracic spine
- Cleanses your lungs, heart, liver and stomach
- Opens the triple heater and small intestine meridians

1 Come into Diamond Pose (Page 84). Raise your arms to shoulder height and bring your right arm across your left above the elbow. Bend your elbow and twist your right arm around your left arm until your palms can be placed together. Your thumbs should point towards your nose.

2 Focus on lengthening through your spine and relaxing your shoulders.

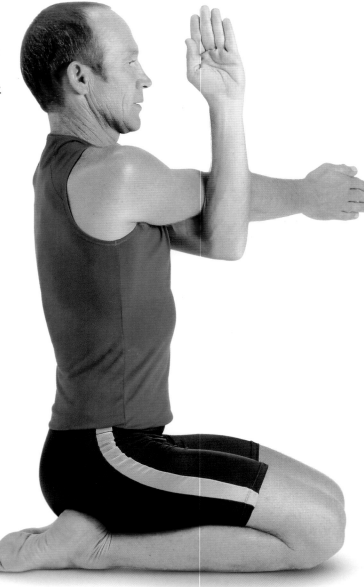

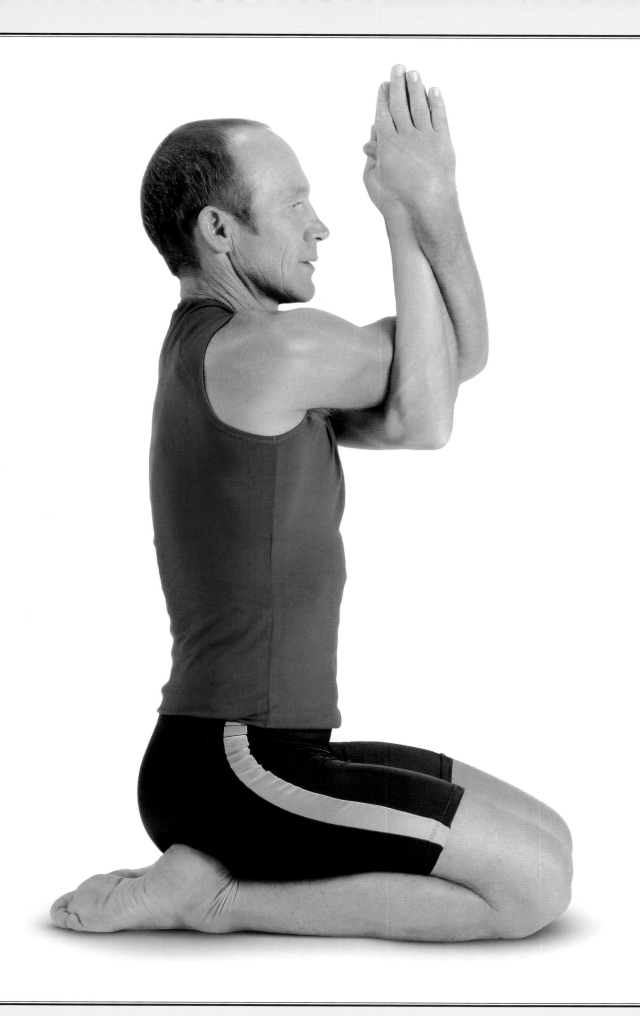

DIAMOND POSE
WITH SHOULDER EXTENSION

Benefits
- Stretches tight ankles and quadriceps. Opens your chest and releases tension in tight shoulders.
- Stretches muscles involved in respiration for better breathing
- Strengthens your heart and lungs.
- Opens your heart, lungs and pericardium meridan

1 Sit in Diamond Pose (Page 84), extend your arms overhead and interlace your fingers as you turn the palms upward. Keep your gaze forward.

2 Relax your shoulders and continue to lengthen your spine upwards.

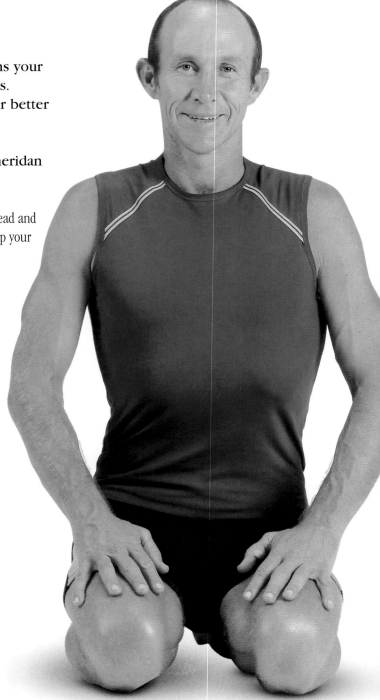

SOFTER
If you have tightness in your joints, place a cushion under your buttocks.

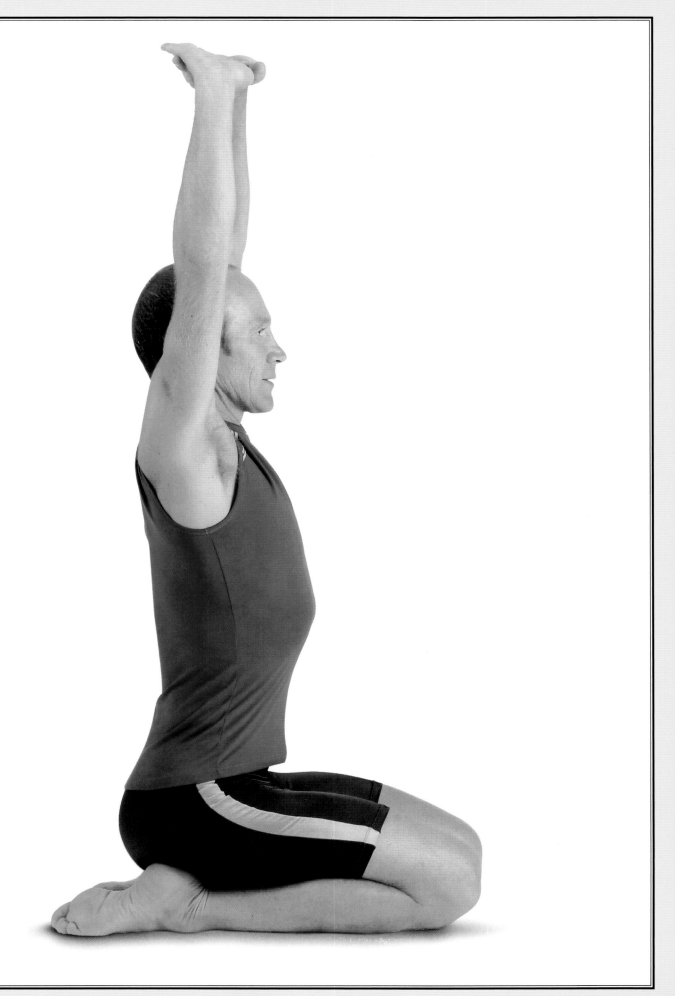

TIGER POSE

VYAGHRASANA

Benefits

- Improves spinal flexibility, relaxes your sciatic nerves
- Tones your abdomen, hips and thighs
- Strengthens your nervous system and activates circulation to all the organs
- Cleanses your colon and lungs
- Opens your bladder meridan

DYNAMIC VERSION

1 Begin on all fours. Extend your right leg back, parallel to the ground. Check your pelvis is stable, bend your right knee and point your toes towards the back of your head. Look downward.

2 Swing the bent leg under your right hip and take your knee toward your chest. Tuck your chin into your chest. Keep your ankle, knee and hip alignment. Continue dynamically 5 times and repeat left side.

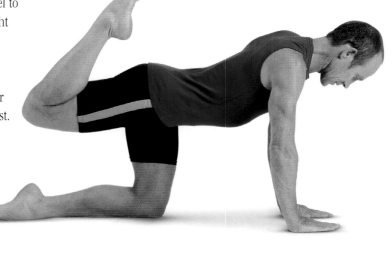

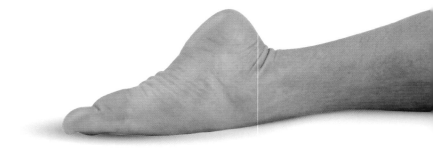

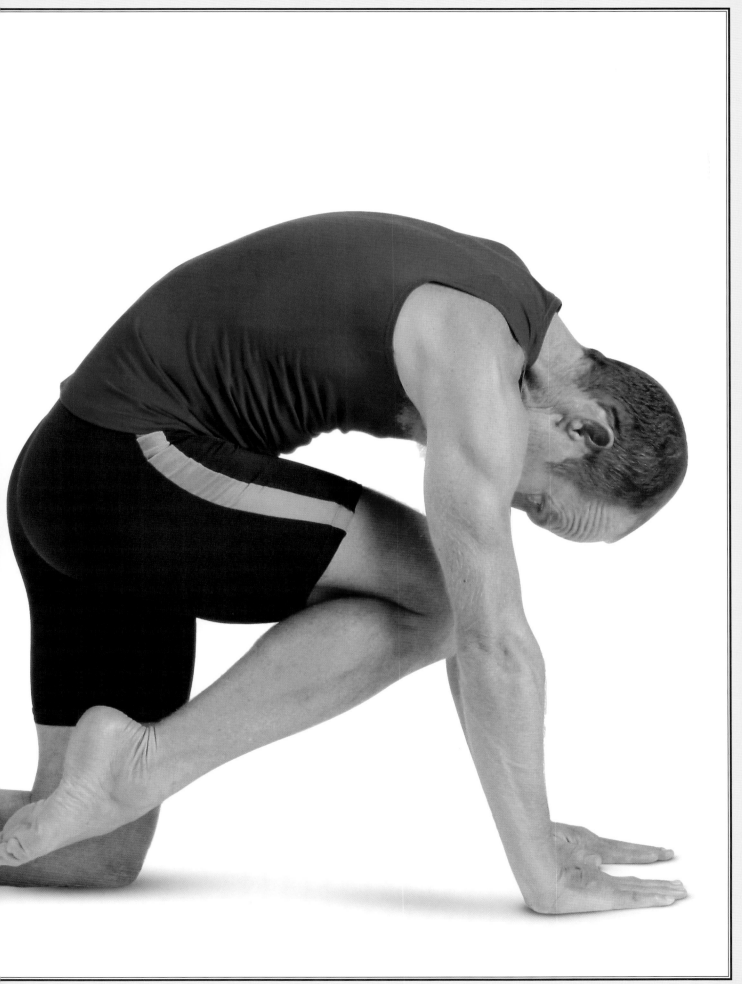

STAFF POSE

DANDASANA

Benefits
- Stretches and extends your spine
- Effective for toning your whole body and helps develop postural strength
- Strengthens your heart and lungs
- Opens your stomach meridian

1 Begin seated, extending to straight legs keeping your knee joints unlocked, feet are hip width apart, toes pointing upwards.

2 Place your hands behind you, palms down, fingers spread, and relax your shoulders.

3 Balance on your sitting bones and lengthen through your spine. Lift your chest and open your heart centre. Hold for 20 seconds. To increase the effectiveness of this pose, keep your spine vertical and retain its natural curve.

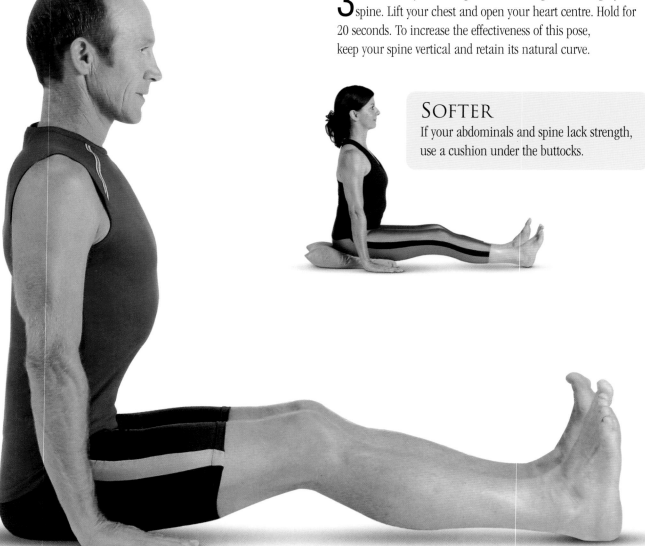

SOFTER
If your abdominals and spine lack strength, use a cushion under the buttocks.

SITTING FORWARD BEND

PASCIMOTTANASANA

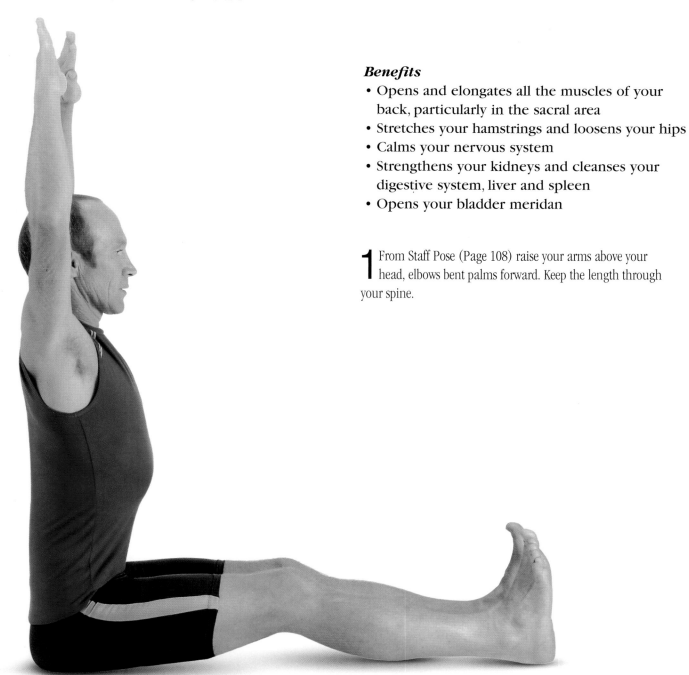

Benefits
- Opens and elongates all the muscles of your back, particularly in the sacral area
- Stretches your hamstrings and loosens your hips
- Calms your nervous system
- Strengthens your kidneys and cleanses your digestive system, liver and spleen
- Opens your bladder meridan

1 From Staff Pose (Page 108) raise your arms above your head, elbows bent palms forward. Keep the length through your spine.

Sitting
Forward Bend

(continued)

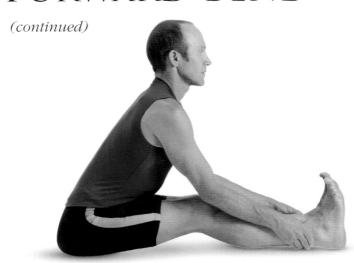

2 Anchor your buttocks and fold forward from your hip joints. Without rounding your spine, rest your hands alongside your shins, ankles or feet.

3 If you have the flexibility, continue to fold forward and rest your head between your shins. Hold for 20 seconds.

4 Return to an upright position by reversing the path taken into the forward bend.

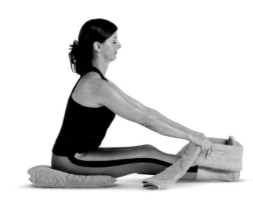

Softer

If your lower back rounds, sit on a cushion so that your hips are raised slightly. Hold a towel around your feet and keep your spine lengthening up and forward.

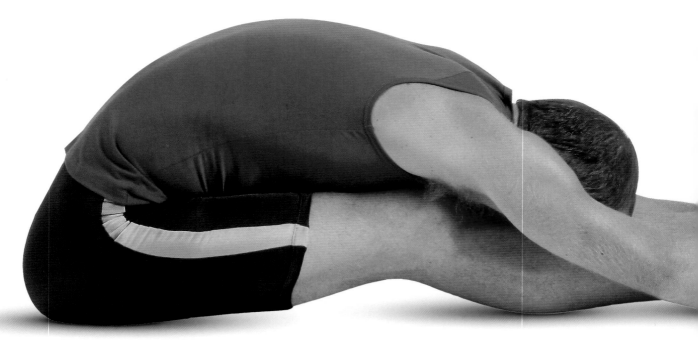

SITTING HALF TWIST

ARDA MATSYENDRASANA

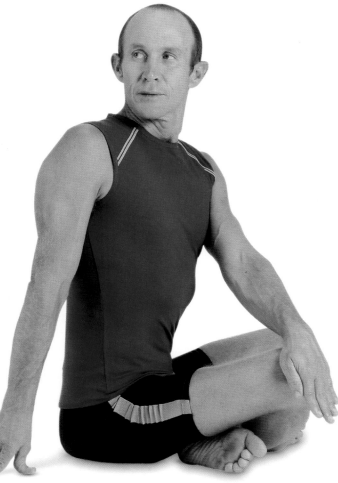

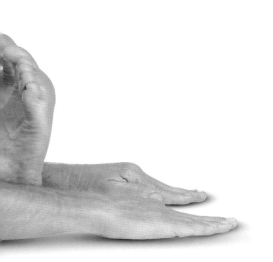

Benefits
- Tones your spinal nerves, makes your back muscles supple and loosens your vertebrae
- Cleanses and massages your digestive system, liver, pancreas, kidneys and spleen
- Opens your gallbladder meridian

1 Sit with your legs crossed and with your back upright. Place your right hand out to the side of your buttocks and come onto your fingertips. Your left hand rests on the outside of your right knee.

2 Extend up through your spine and head. Stabilise your pelvis and twist to the right commencing from the lumber spine and continuing up. Keep your shoulders level throughout.

3 Continue to lengthen your spine. Hold for 10 seconds and repeat opposite side

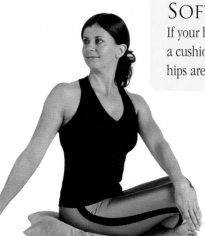

SOFTER
If your back is not straight, sit on a cushion throughout so that your hips are raised slightly.

CROCODILE TWIST

JATHARA PARIVARTANASANA

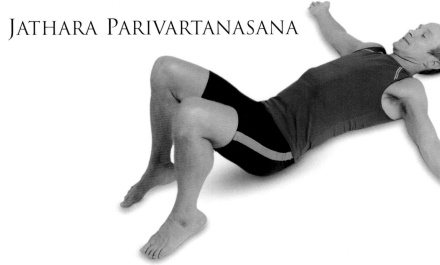

Benefits
- Stretches your lower back and sciatic nerves. Relieves backache
- Aligns your spinal vertebrae
- Cleanses your digestive system, liver and gallbladder
- Opens your gallbladder meridian

1 Lie on your back with your arms outstretched at shoulder height, palms up. Bend your knees and place your soles on the ground a little wider than hip width apart. Relax your abdomen.

DYNAMIC VERSION

2 Lower your knees to the right and look towards your left shoulder. Keep both feet and shoulders in contact with the ground. Bring your knees back to centre then alternate to the left, and look towards your right hand. Continue dynamically for 45 seconds.

STATIC VERSION

3 Hold the twist for 10 seconds each side and return your legs to centre.

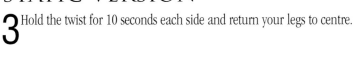

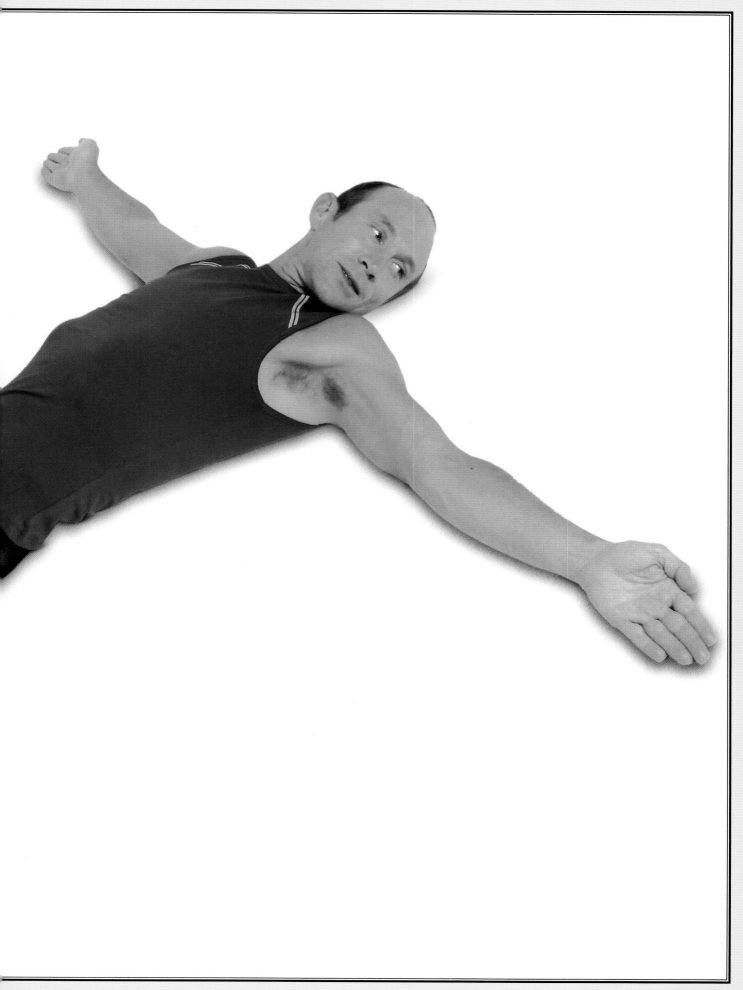

KNEE TO CHEST POSE

Benefits
- Opens your hips
- Stretches your lower back and sciatic nerves
- Massages your abdominal organs
- Opens your bladder meridian

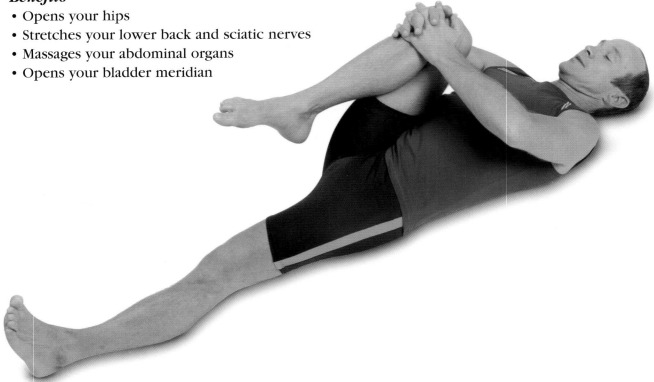

1 Lying on your back, bring your right leg up. Interlace your fingers below your knee and take your knee to chest.

2 Keep your chin tucked and spine extended. Hold for 10 seconds, and continue into Lever Pose (Page 115, steps 1→3). Repeat with your left leg.

LEVER POSE

Benefits
- Helps relieve backache
- Opens your lower thoracic and lumber spine
- Gives a gentle squeeze to your abdominal organs and helps peristalsis in your intestines
- Increases a sense of vitality
- Opens your bladder and gallbladder meridian

1 Place your left hand on the outside of your right knee. Extend your right arm out from your shoulder (palms up).

2 Relax your abdomen and lower your right knee to the left. Look at your right hand. Hold for 10 seconds.

3 Return your leg to the centre and extend out straight.

4 Repeat with your left leg, Knee to Chest Pose (Page 115) then above steps 1–3.

5 Come into Womb Pose (Page 118) as a counter pose.

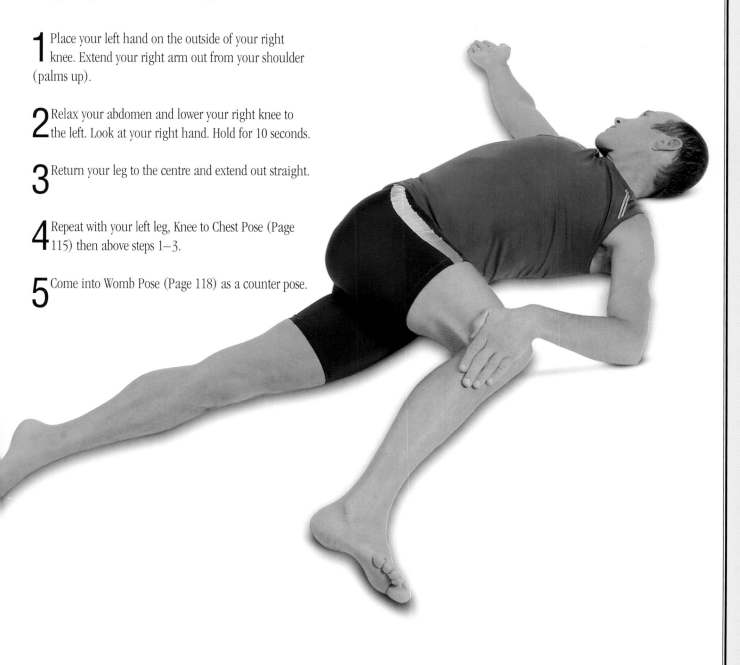

HALF BRIDGE

SETU BANKHA SARVANANGASANA

Benefits
- Stretches and massages your colon and other abdominal organs
- Stretches the front of your hips, increasing flexibility
- Nourishes your thyroid gland with a fresh blood supply
- Strengthens your lungs, heart, liver, spleen, stomach and cleanses your kidneys and spine
- Opens your stomach meridian

1 Lie on your back. Bring your feet up towards your buttocks as far as they will comfortably go. Place your feet hip width apart. Place your arms at your side, palms down. Lengthen through your spine and keep your chin slightly tucked in.

DYNAMIC VERSION

2 Begin by pressing down on the floor with your feet and slowly raise your hips. Feel one vertebra at a time peeling off the floor. The weight of your body is equally supported by your feet, shoulders, and arms. Keep your chest lifting and opening, and legs parallel.

3 Return to lying on your back by reversing the motion. Move very slowly replacing vertebra by vertebra onto the ground. Rest with the back of your abdomen flat on the ground. Repeat 3 times holding the third bridge statically.

STATIC VERSION

4 Hold the bridge keeping your feet and shoulders stationary. Keep your shoulders relaxed and chin tucked in. Hold for 10 seconds and return to starting position.

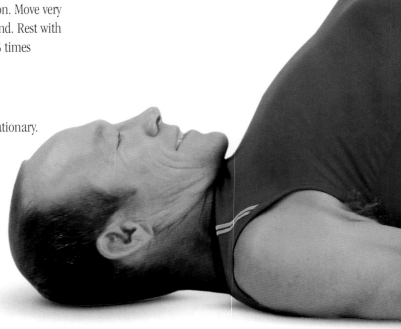

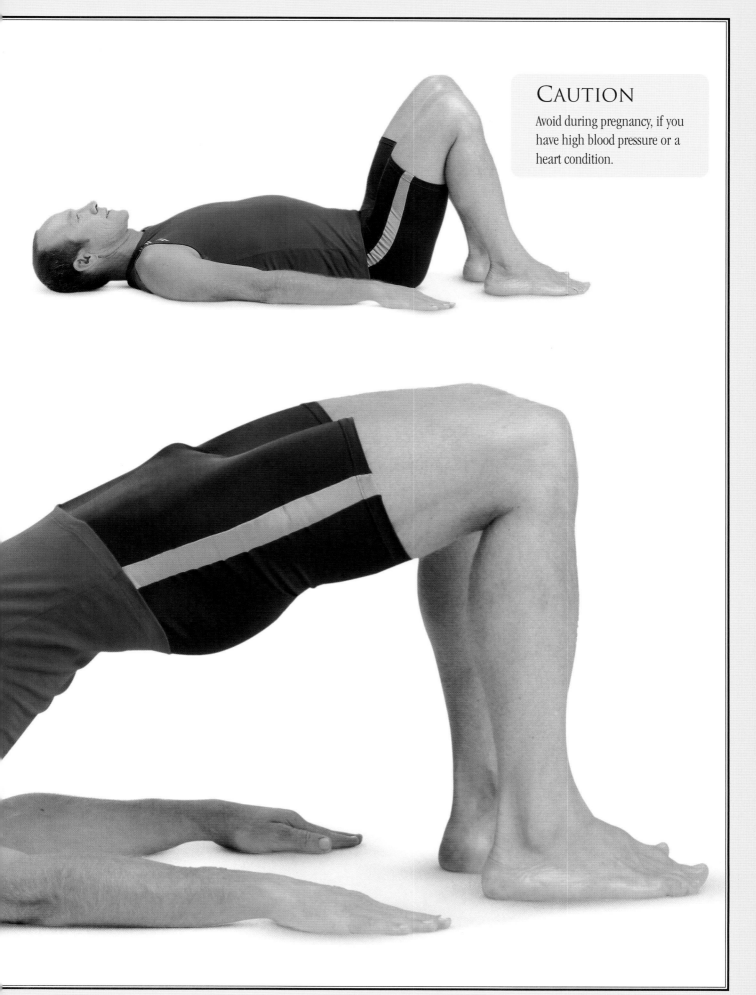

CAUTION

Avoid during pregnancy, if you have high blood pressure or a heart condition.

WOMB POSE

ASPANASANA

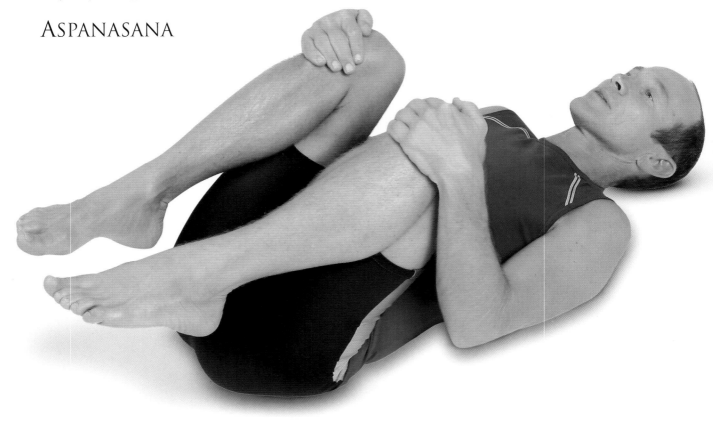

Benefits
- Stretches your lower back and hips
- Stretches your sciatic nerves
- Excellent for digestion, massaging your large and small intestine
- Counter posture to backbends, twist and strong standing postures

1 Lie on your back, bend one leg up at a time, holding below your knee take your thighs into your abdomen. Keep your knees hip width apart and relax your neck and shoulders. Elongate through the back of your neck, keeping your chin tucked in. Hold for 20 seconds.

2 Return to starting position by extending out one leg at a time.

BIRTH POSE

Benefits

- Stretches your groin and hips
- Increases circulation to your pelvic cavity
- Strengthens your kidneys, uterus and genitals
- Opens your kidney, liver and spleen meridians

1 Lie on your back and bring your feet towards your buttocks until comfortable. Place your arms at your side, palms up. Join the soles together and slowly allow your knees to fall outwards, towards the earth. Allow the natural arch to remain in the spine. Close your eyes and observe the rhythmic flow of breath below your navel. Hold for 60 seconds.

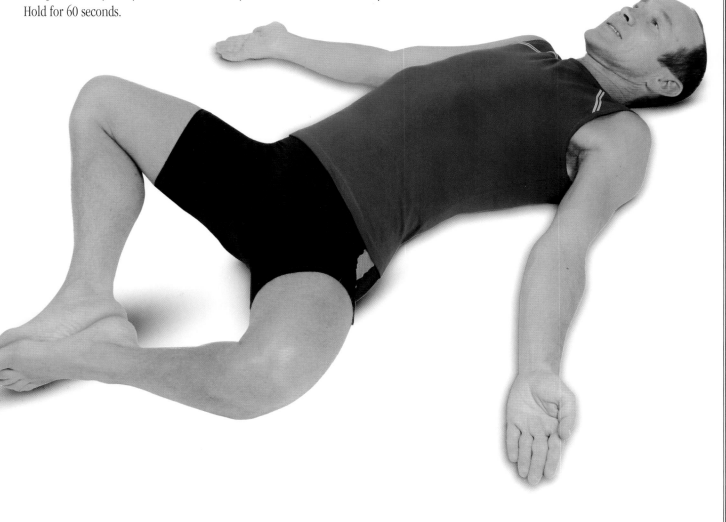

PEACEFUL POSE

SHAVASANA

Benefits
- Relaxes your whole body and mind
- A counter posture to all the previous Asanas
- Allows you to fully absorb the energy that has been released and accumulated throughout the *Yoga Class*
- During relaxation your body can recuperate, repair and rejuvenate itself
- An opportunity to surrender any resistance, let go and 'be at peace'

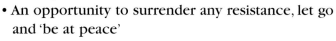

1 Repeat steps 1 to 3 (Page 76). Remain in Peaceful Pose for 5 minutes or longer.

2 Bring your awareness back to your body giving your toes and fingers a wriggle. Keeping your eyes closed bend your right leg, then left. Roll to your right side and come up to sitting cross-legged.

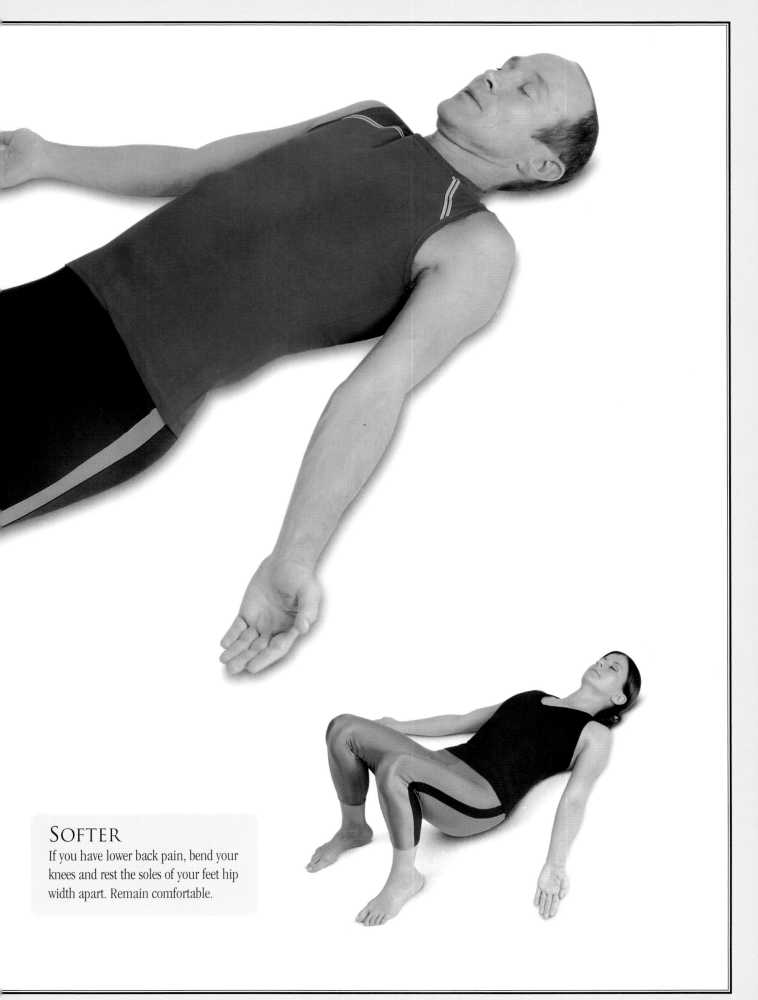

SOFTER
If you have lower back pain, bend your knees and rest the soles of your feet hip width apart. Remain comfortable.

PRAYER POSE
SITTING CROSS LEGGED WITH HANDS IN PRAYER POSE
DHYANA

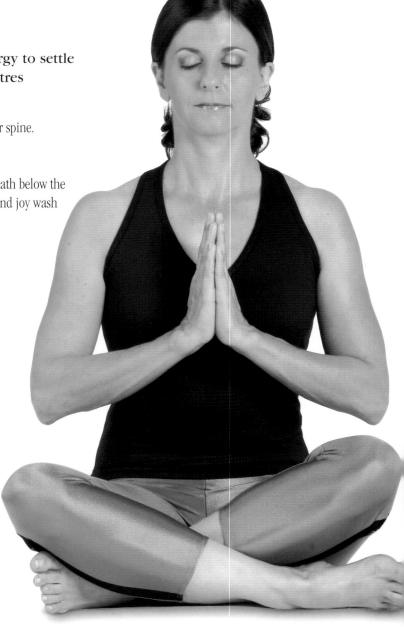

Benefits
- A concluding posture to allow your energy to settle
- Integrates your thinking and feeling centres

1 Sit cross-legged with your eyes closed. Lengthen your spine.

2 Bring your hands into Prayer Pose. Be with your breath below the navel for a few moments. Feel a sense of calmness and joy wash down through your body. Slowly open your eyes.

'NAMASTE'

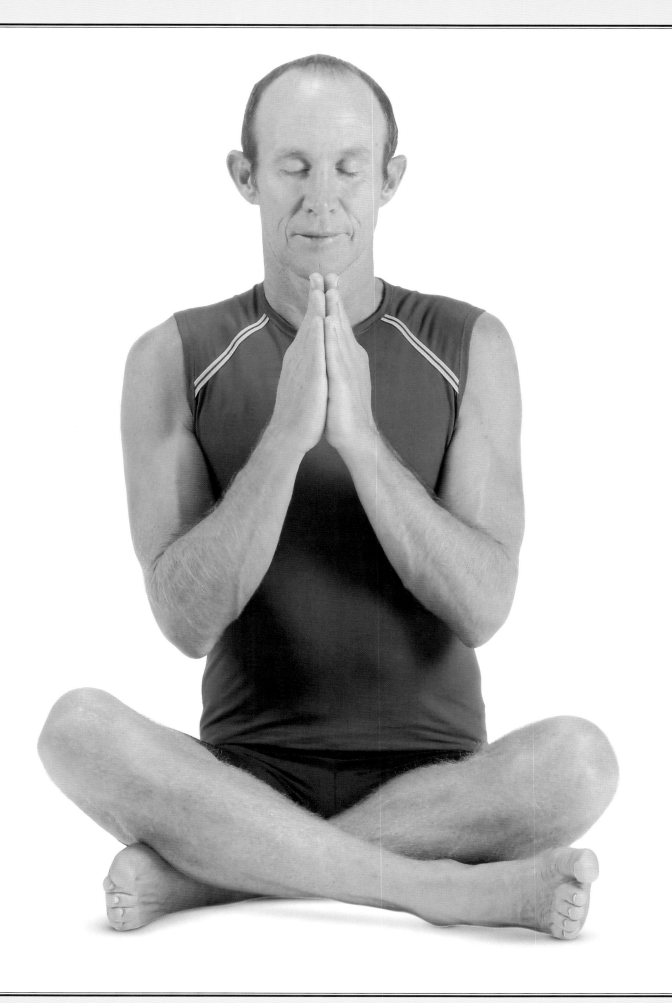

LET FOOD BE YOUR MEDICINE

To gain the most out of Yoga, certain awareness must also be placed on what we put into our bodies. Unfortunately over the years our Western dietary choices have placed most peoples' health on 'Red Alert'. From an early age, we are brought up on a diet of commercially packaged, de-vitalized and nutrient-deficient foods. This leaves our bodies depleted of vitamins and minerals, and vulnerable to many illnesses. Fortunately, through the right dietary choices, we can begin to provide our bodies with the nutrients it requires for better health and longevity. This will also benefit our bodies and mind to become more balanced, throughout your yoga practice.

Traditional medicine is based on the premise that there is a self regulating, self healing power within each person, and when the correct nutrients and conditions are provided, the human body is able to heal itself.

A healthy diet is one which is enjoyable and nutritious. The primary reason for eating food is to nourish the body and produce life energy (Chi). It is abundant in whole 'natural' and unprocessed foods. It is especially high in plant foods, such as fruits, vegetables, grains, beans, seeds and nuts.

FOOD AS MEDICINE

Plants absorb minerals from the soil and water. Through the action of photosynthesis they manufacture vitamins, fatty acids, carbohydrates and proteins. Unfortunately, at times, even if we are complying with a healthy diet, our body is not getting its nutritional requirements met. This may be attributed to poor digestion and assimilation, mineral deficient soils, monocrop farming, use of insecticides and herbicides, air and water pollution. The way food is transported, stored and processed also diminishes it nutrient value, especially its vitamin content.

To ensure your body is receiving optimum health and nutritional requirements, 'Super Foods' – high in natural vitamins, minerals, essential fatty acids, proteins, enzymes and antioxidants – should be considered.

SUPERFOODS

- **Spirulina, Wheat grass, Green Barley Powder**
  Contains 98 out of 100 earth elements. Rich in chlorophyll, which bears a close resemblance to haemoglobin.

- **Vegetable Juice**
  Carrot, beetroot, celery and ginger. A wonderful elixir to cleanse the body. Contains a wide spectrum of vitamins, enzymes and alkalizing minerals.

- **Fatty Acids**
  Equal portions of olive and linseed with a small portion of wheat germ oil. Gives the body its requirements of Omega 3 and Omega 6 essential fatty acids.

- **Seaweed/Kelp Powder**
  One of the most nutritious foods on the earth. High in minerals, especially trace minerals, vitamin B12.

- **Pollen Granules**
  A rich natural source of amino acids. Recognized as a complete food.

- **Royal Maca**
  A natural phytoestrogen. Rich in minerals and trace minerals.

- **Rosehip Powder**
  High in natural Vitamin C and minerals.

DIGESTION ROUTINE

To improve digestion, the following postures can be practised after a meal. Begin with:

- Peaceful Pose (Page 76)
- The Main Central Energy Series (Page 84–91)
- Crocodile Twist (Page 112)
- Womb Pose (Page 118)
- Peaceful Pose (Page 76)

Certain kinds of foods may also influence the body and mind in ways that are either beneficial or detrimental to health. This may depend on the individuals Ayurvedic type or blood type. The importance of correct food-combining of major food groups, such as proteins and carbohydrates, fruit and vegetables also needs to be addressed. For more specific personal advice contact your closest Ayurvedic Naturopath or Health Care Practitioner.

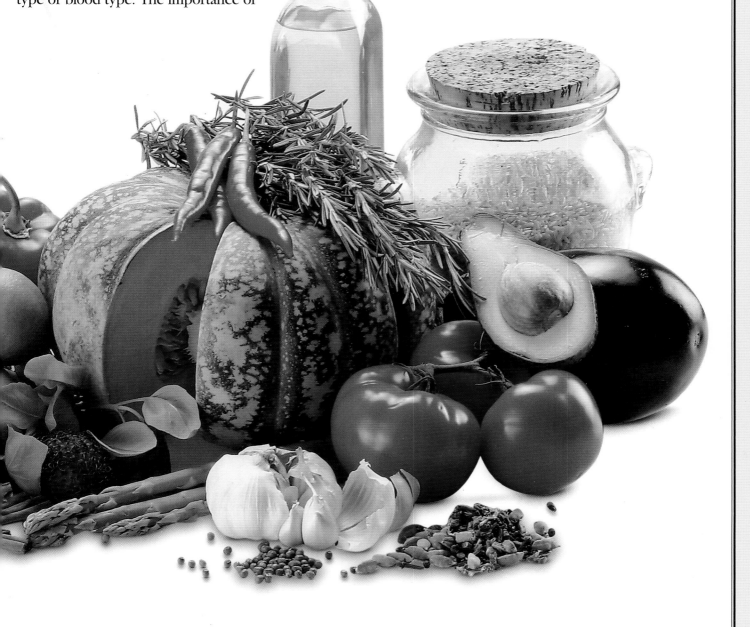

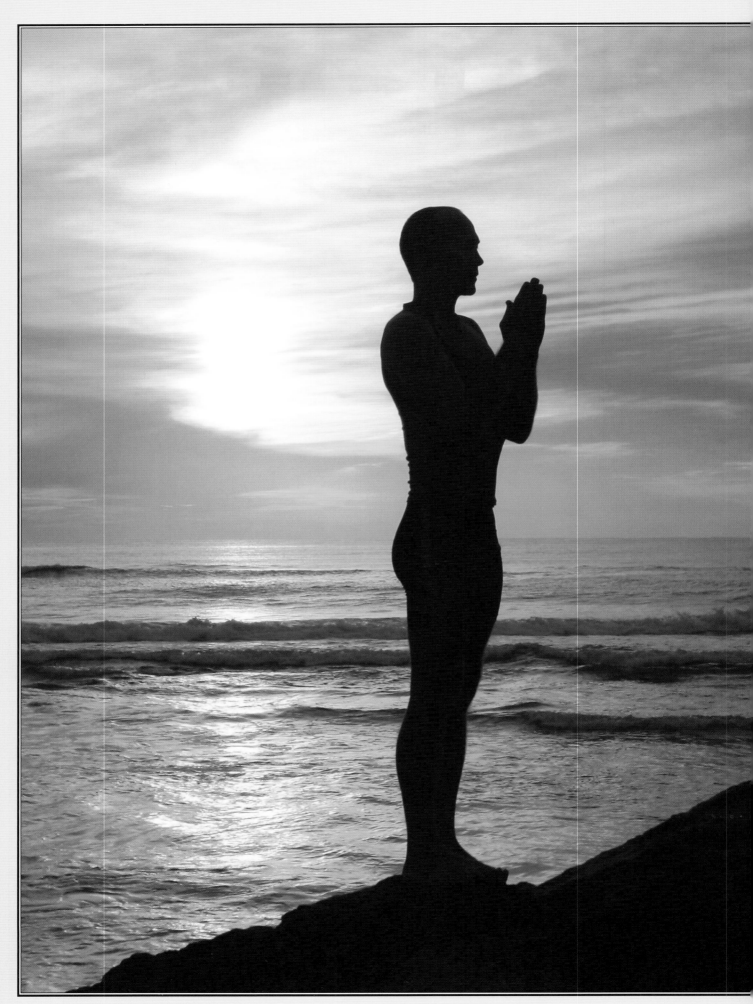

GLOSSARY

ASANA
A yoga posture, a combination of physical alignment and mental awareness

AYURVEDA
Traditional healing system of India. It is a complete health system for mind, body and spirit. Works holistically to prevent and treat disease.

CEREBROSPINAL FLUID
Plasma-like fluid that fills the cavities of the central nervous system.

CERVICAL
The neck.

CHI
Life force, energy.

CHI GUNG
A collective term for various arts that develop energy for health, martial arts, mental training and spiritual development.

CHLOROPHYLL
The green pigment of plants that traps the energy of sunlight.

CONNECTIVE TISSUE
A primary tissue. Functions include support, storage and protection.

DIAPHRAGM
Dome-shaped skeletal muscle between the thoracic and abdominal cavities.

DYNAMIC VERSION
A continuous movement throughout a posture. Circulates energy.

ENDOCRINE SYSTEM
Body system that includes internal organs that secrete hormones.

FASCIA
Layers of fibrous tissue covering and separating muscles.

HATHA
Refers to the balance of male and female. When applied, brings the two sides of the body into balance.

HAEMOGLOBIN
A substance in red blood cells, involved in the transport of oxygen and carbon dioxide.

LATERAL
Relating to the side or sides.

LUMBAR SPINE
Portion of the back between the thorax and the pelvis.

MAIN CENTRAL ENERGY
A circular flow of energy commencing from the base, up the back, and down the front of the body. It is made up of the governing (yang) and conception (ying) vessels.

MERIDIANS
Pathways of energy flow in the body.

PHYTOESTROGEN
A plant molecule that regulates the body's natural estrogen.

PRANA
Life force, life energy.

SACRUM
The large wedge shape bone in the lower part of the back.

SCIATIC NERVES
Two nerves that descend from the lower back through the thigh down the back of the legs.

STATIC VERSION
Holding a posture. Directs energy.

SYMPATHETIC NERVOUS SYSTEM
Primarily concerned with the processes involving the expenditure of energy, i.e. 'fight' or 'flight' response.

THORACIC
The part of the body enclosed by the ribs.

VESSELS
Pathways of energy flow in the body.

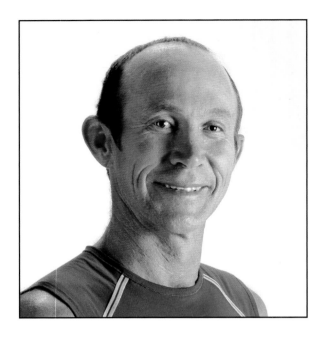

About the Author

GARY BROMLEY

Gary Bromley is a highly experienced practitioner in the field of Natural Therapies.

He is involved in the study and practice of Yoga, Chi Gung, Naturopathy and Ayurvedic Medicine – a traditional healing system.

A passionate believer in 'Preventative Medicine', Gary has created his own totally natural health-care range using only 100% natural ingredients.

A special understanding of natural medicine and it's health benefits, has enabled Gary to provide a health care program tailored specifically to suit each individual, which in turn attracts clients to his health clinic on the Gold Coast in Queensland, Australia.

He will offer you a warm welcome, and be happy to answer your questions about *Yoga Class*.

YOGA

One Partner-Sharing
& One Individual
—Yoga Class—

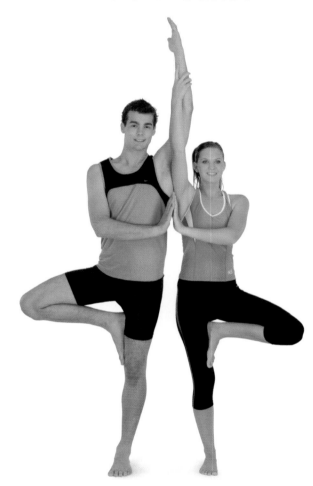

Author: Lynley Woods
Art Director: Karen Moores
Editor: Jane Keighley
Graphic Artist: Melissa Carroll
Photographer: Glenn Weiss
Special thanks to models Sarah Burgess
and Matthew Dezoete-Baker

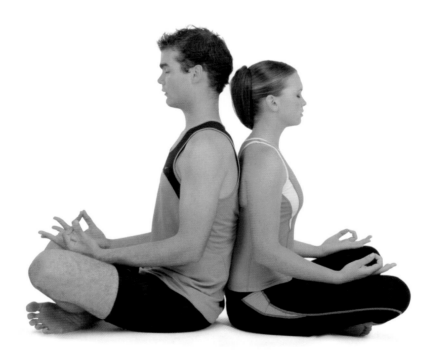

CONTENTS

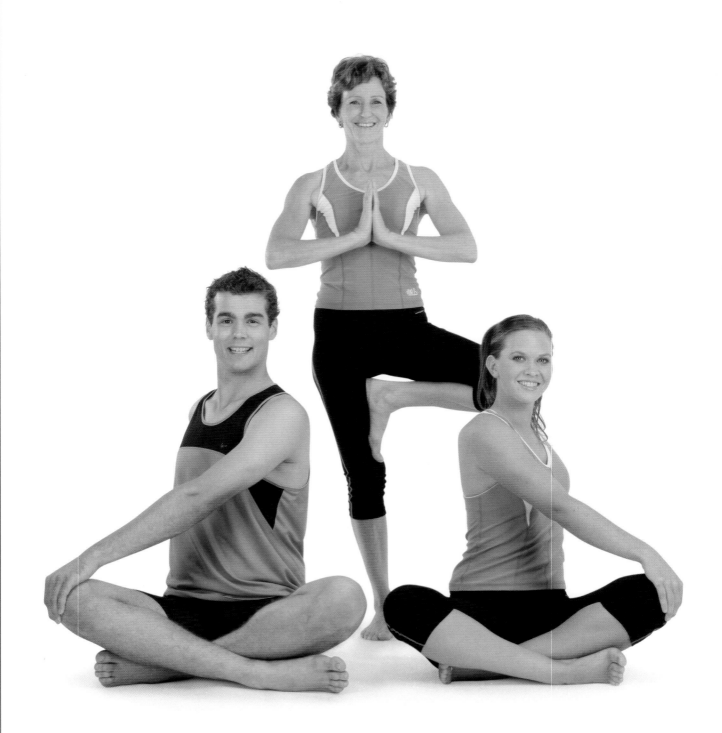

INTRODUCTION TO YOGA

Practising yoga can give the experience of lightness, release and joy. No-one is too young or too old to try it, because there are so many facets to this ancient, holistic life science. The word 'yoga' is derived from Sanskrit, one of the oldest known languages. It has a twofold meaning:

1 the verb, to bind or yoke, implying steady, consistent practise, and;

2 the noun, union, denoting the harmonising of all aspects of our being – body, mind and spirit.

The form of yoga with which most Westerners are familiar is hatha (the union of ha – the masculine sun and tha – the feminine moon). It's a unique blend of physical postures (asana), breath control (pranayama) and relaxation (or sense withdrawal – pratyahara).

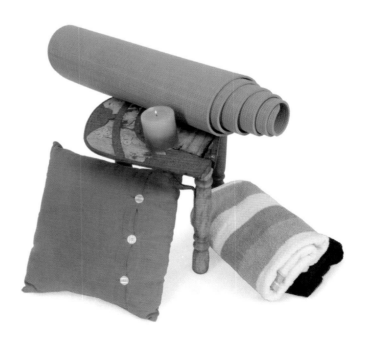

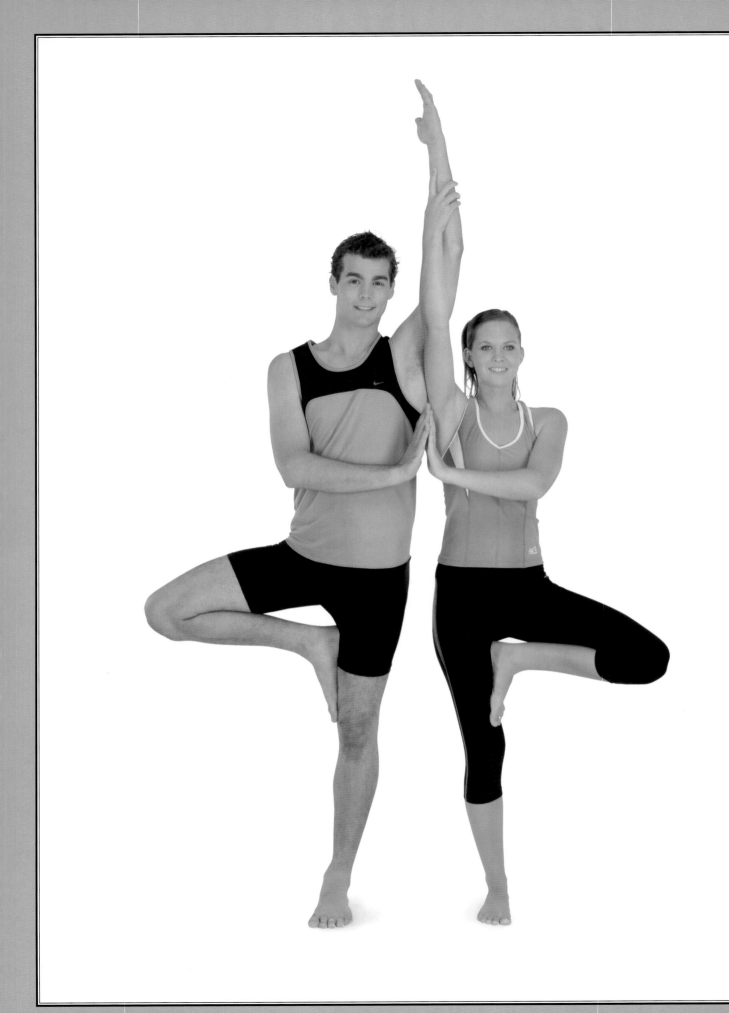

BENEFITS

More than just a set of physical exercises, this combination promotes health, flexibility, strength, vitality, endurance and wellbeing on all levels – physical, emotional and mental. The physical benefits alone are a good incentive for practising yoga, which

- Strengthens, tones and revitalises your musculoskeletal system

- Cleanses, tones and maintains your vital organs, blood and lymph circulation

- Improves the functioning of your endocrine system, regulating the efficient production of hormones throughout your body

The control and co-ordination of your breath with the postures, along with the mental focus applied, gives the ability to stabilise and calm your mind and emotions, improving mental clarity and efficiency. People often find while practising yoga that they experience a cleansing effect, resulting in a feeling of lightness and an increase of energy. This can further inspire lifestyle changes including:

- An improvement in diet – reducing or eliminating refined and processed foods and replacing them with fresh, natural whole foods which increase the intake of life force (prana)

- Spending more time in fresh air and natural surroundings

GOING DEEPER

Even further, there can be the incentive for looking into the deeper levels of yoga. The ancient sages tell us that we are actually spiritual beings having a human experience for a short time on earth.

Our true essence is one of light and joy, and we can connect with that essence by taking some time to withdraw from our worldly concerns, allowing our mind to slow down and move into silence.

The realisation of our true nature and potential enables us to lead more enriching lives, and to feel happier and more complete. That state of inner-peace has a positive effect on our behaviour and ultimately our relationships with people, our community and the environment.

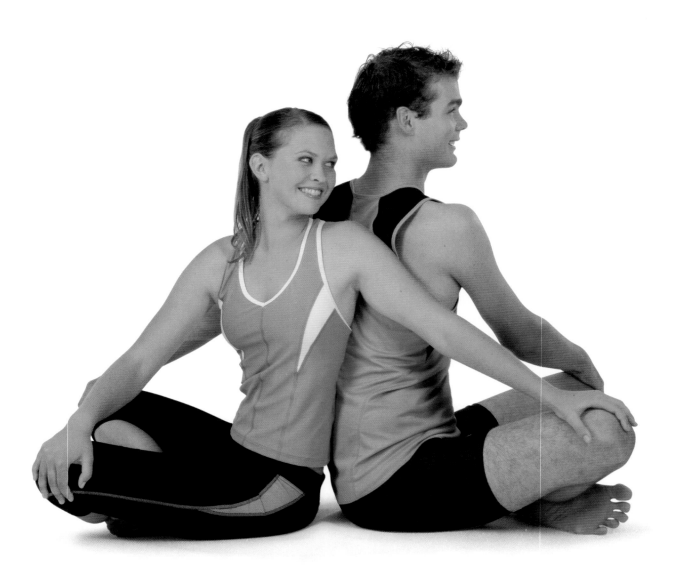

ABOUT PARTNER-SHARING & INDIVIDUAL YOGA

Partner-Sharing & Individual Yoga has three sections:

1 A general class.

2 An added section of partner-assisted postures.

3 A guided relaxation.

If you are new to yoga, there are gentler variations of the more difficult postures, allowing scope for progress. If you are familiar with it, *Partner-Sharing and Individual Yoga* can add variety to your practise.

SUGGESTED GUIDELINES

1 Yoga is ideally practised slowly with body awareness and co-ordinated breathing.

2 Never force yourself into a position. Work to the best of your ability but relax. This will make the stretches easier and open your mind to experience the benefits. If you want to create a challenge, learn the difference between discomfort and pain. A little discomfort is fine in order to make progress. Strain or pain is the body's signal to back off.

3 Yoga stimulates the metabolism and enhances the effects of whatever is consumed. If taking prescribed medication (or you have ANY injuries or medical conditions) consult a medical practitioner first.

4 Postures are best practised on an empty stomach, so first thing in the morning is ideal. But find a time that suits your lifestyle, where you can be undisturbed and relaxed, in order to benefit from the centring effects of yoga.

5 Practise in a clean, airy space, one that preferably enhances feelings of wellbeing. You don't need a large area. If you don't have a yoga mat, a carpeted area or a non-slip rug will do. Keep a cushion and blanket close by in case you need them. Clothing should be unrestricted to allow ease of movement and feet kept bare.

6 Read through this book, taking note of the cautions, before you start practising.

YOGA PHILOSOPHY

Many people regard yoga as a religion. This is not the case. It is a simple, practical philosophy that does not conflict with, or contradict, any existing religion. As numerous practitioners attest, yoga complements and enriches anyone's personal beliefs. Originally, the teachings were passed on from teacher to student by word of mouth. Somewhere around the 2nd or 3rd centuries BC, a learned sage by the name of Patanjali codified the yoga philosophy into written form.

He stated that:

- The aim of yoga is "stilling the fluctuations of the mind"

- These fluctuations are controlled through consistent practise and detachment (not clinging to the results of the practise, but letting them evolve)

- Enlightenment will result from practising the 8 limbs of yoga

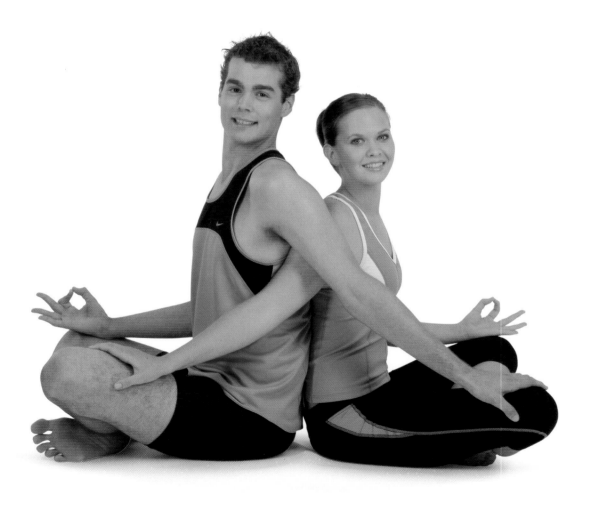

The 8 Limbs

1 Restraints in our dealings with the external world (yamas).

2 Observances for our personal self (niyamas).

3 Postures (asana).

4 Breath control (pranayama).

5 Sense withdrawal (pratyahara).

6 Concentration (dharana).

7 Meditation (dhyana).

8 Pure consciousness (samadhi).

The last 6 limbs have been introduced in other sections of this book, so following is a brief description of the first 2 limbs which define the ethics and morals of yoga.

Restraints (Yamas)

1 Harmlessness, non-violence – in thought and word as well as deed, basic consideration and respect.

2 Truthfulness, non-lying – to self as well as others.

3 Non-theft – of energy and time, as well as on the material level.

4 Moderation of the senses and appetites – realising the difference between need and indulgence.

5 Non-greed, non-attachment – separating needs from wants, non-possessive, non-selfish.

Observances (Niyamas)

1 Cleanliness – purity in mind and body, inner and outer.

2 Contentment – acceptance, gratitude, equanimity.

3 Committed focus – integrity of motive, willingness, taking personal responsibility.

4 Self-study – awareness of motives and actions, uplifting readings.

5 Attentiveness to God – whatever you conceive a higher power to be, to nurture your spirit.

These were presented as limbs rather than steps as they can be practised separately or as a whole and in no particular order. It is believed that all humans long for wholeness, unity and completion, so practising one or a few of these limbs will result in integrating all of them in the long run.

YOGA & BREATHING

The yoga sages taught that the breath contains prana (life force). By developing the awareness of our natural breath first and then advancing to various control techniques (pranayama), we can enhance and direct the flow and effect of this precious life force.

For example, during the postures if there is discomfort in a certain area, by consciously exhaling into that area we can experience a release of tension making it possible to relax more into the pose.

The breath in yoga is seen as a bridge between the body and the mind and also between the mind and the spirit – the grand unifier.

By focusing on the flow of the breath it can become a tool for concentration (dharana) enabling the mind to develop stillness and one-pointedness (meditation – dhyana). Once this state is reached it is possible for a subtle transformation to occur – a spontaneous feeling of wholeness and union with all that there is (samadhi).

HUMMING BEE BREATH
BHRAMARI

This simple technique may be used at the beginning or end of your posture work to calm and centre your mind.

Benefits
- Physical – the vibration relieves any blockages and problems of your nasal and ear passages such as sinus and tinnitus, as well as your throat and upper chest, and may also relieve headaches
- Mental – calms and quiets your mind, especially when anxious or unable to sleep
- An excellent preparation for meditation

1 Sit in an easy position where your back is straight with shoulders, face and jaw relaxed. Breathe in and out through your nose at all times.

2 Breathe in normally. Block ears with index fingers. Breathe out and hum. Try to keep your breath even and flowing smoothly.

3 Repeat this a few times and then relax. Observe the stillness and clarity of your mind.

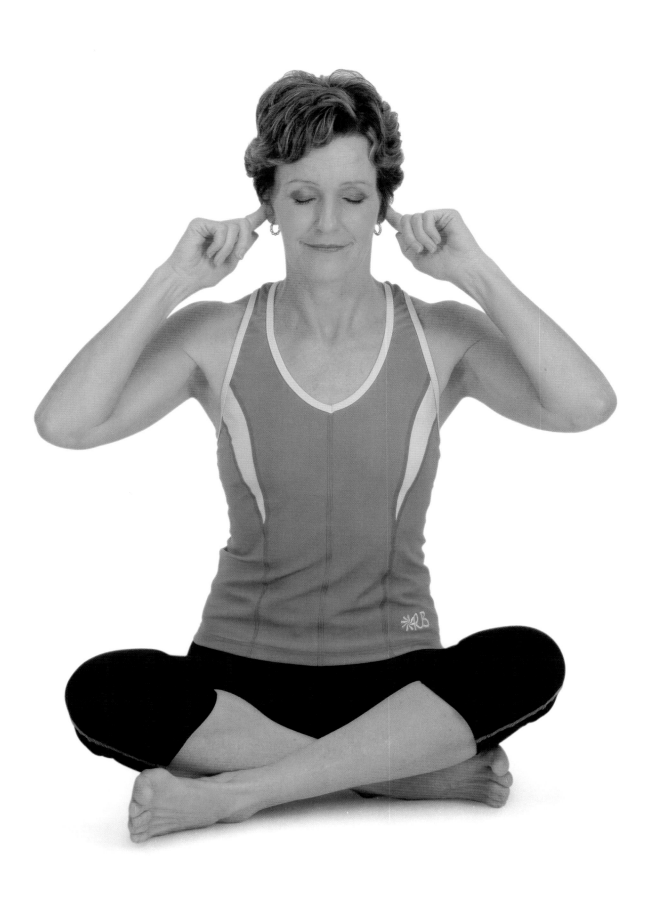

MOUNTAIN POSE

TADASANA

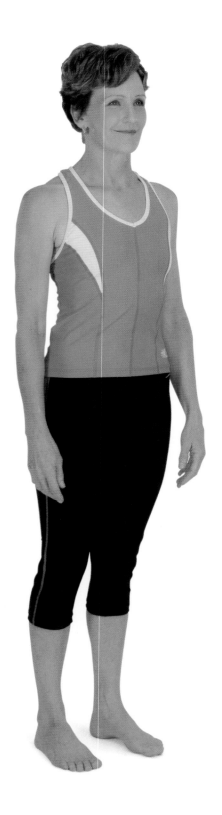

Benefits

- Aligns the whole of your body
- Frees up energy blocks
- Allows efficient function of your organs and nervous and circulatory systems
- Allows full flow of your breath
- Corrects poor postural habits

1 Position feet slightly apart, toes facing forward so feet are parallel and in line. Keep your weight evenly distributed over your feet and feel grounded and connected to the earth. Legs are straight without locking into your knees.

2 Take time to align your hips. Top of pelvic rim is level with the floor and hips not tilted too far forward or back. An internal stretch of your tailbone towards the floor lightly firms your lower abdomen. Lift your heart centre, creating space in the centre of your body.

3 Shoulders are broad and relaxed as if placed on a coathanger. Arms and hands are loose and relaxed.

4 Keep your chin level with the floor to avoid compressing your neck. Have a light internal stretch from your heart centre through the crown of your head towards the heavens. Relax your face and allow it to soften. Either close your eyes or soften your gaze.

5 Focus on your breath, the prana (life force) within the breath, and the free-flow of energy.

IMPORTANT NOTE

Postures have been shown in this book leading to the left. However for regular practice, it is preferable to start on your right side.

LIMBERING

ROTATING TWIST

Benefits

- Warms and loosens up your whole body
- Rhythmical movement calms your nervous system
- Activates both hemispheres of your brain creating mental clarity

1 Position feet hip width apart, facing forward and parallel. Keep knees slightly bent.

2 Turn hips from side-to-side allowing your upper body and arms to passively follow the movement. Keep feet firmly planted so you achieve maximum benefit of the movement through your legs.

3 Keep arms and upper body relaxed so the swinging motion releases your shoulders and neck. Keep your head in line with your spine to avoid excess rotation of your neck.

4 Turn your eyes as far to the side as you can — a nice eye exercise. Keep movement going for 30 to 60 seconds.

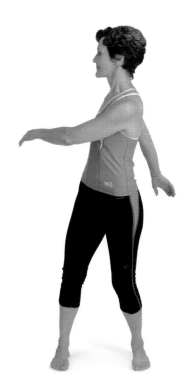
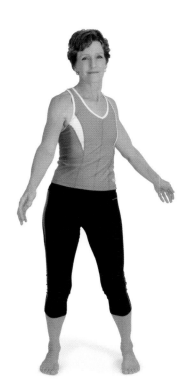
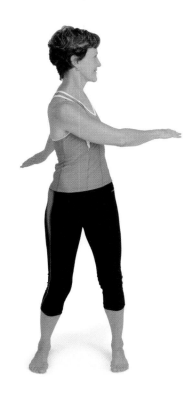

ROLL SHOULDERS

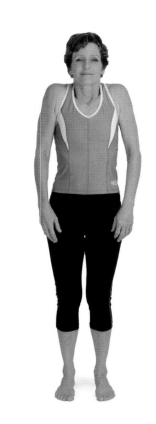

1 Slowly roll shoulders up and back on an inbreath.
Down and forward on an outbreath.

2 Keep head, neck and body stationary.

3 Reverse the movement, 6 times
in each direction.

LOOSEN NECK

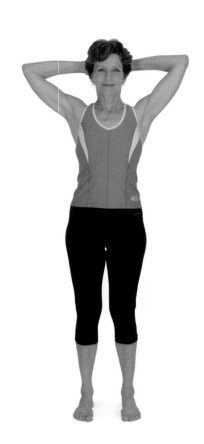

1 Lower head forward and gently shake it from side-to-side. Deepen the
movement bringing your chin up towards one shoulder, down to the centre,
then back up towards your other shoulder. Hold head forward in the centre.
Clasp hands behind your head allowing elbows to fold around your face. Hold
for 5 to 6 breaths, allowing the weight of your hands to gently stretch your neck.

2 Breathe in. Return head upright with hands still behind your head.
Open elbows out wide. Keep chin low and press the back of your head
against your hands. Hold, breathing in and out, then release.

3 Bring one palm to your forehead and press against each other.
Hold for a breath and release.

4 Draw shoulders up in a shrug. Gently shake your head from side-to-side,
massaging neck against your upper shoulder muscles.

5 Turn head to one side and draw your chin down towards your shoulder.
Lift and return back towards your shoulder. Keep shoulders still.
Lift head to centre then lower your ear towards your shoulder and shake your
head gently as if saying no. Return to centre and repeat on the other side.

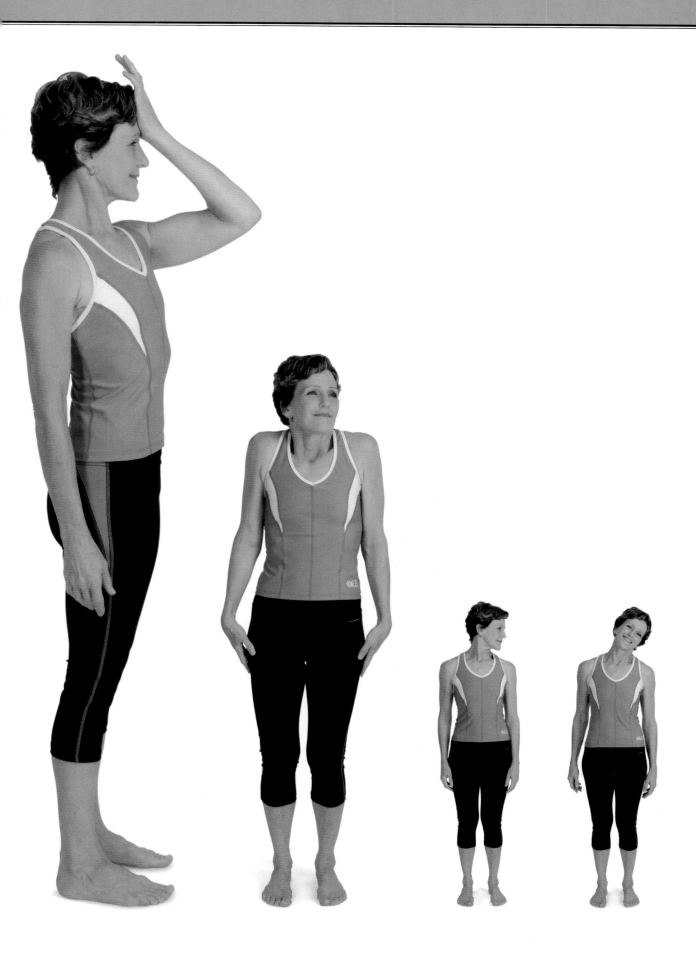

SKI

1 Rock up on your toes, then back on your heels.

2 Use your upper body and arms as if skiing to keep centre of gravity stable. This works all the joints from your toes up through your legs.

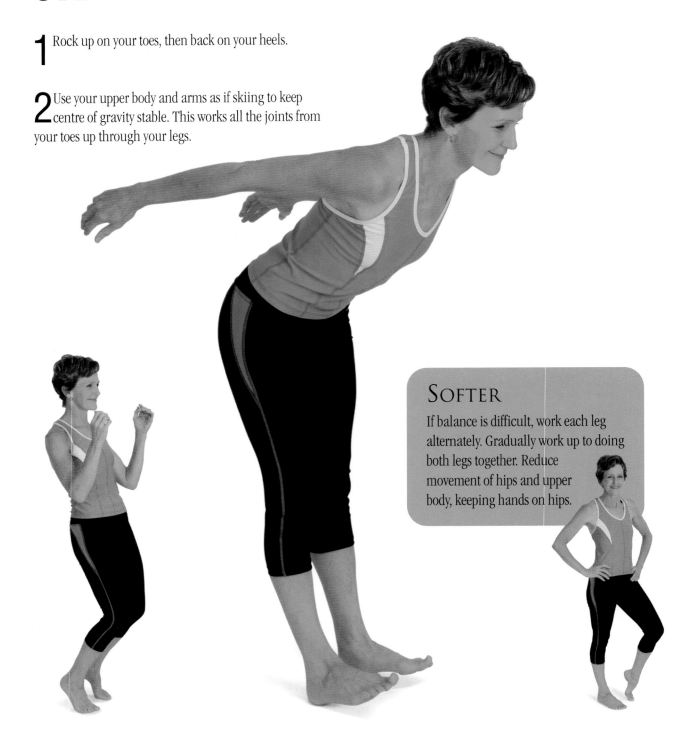

SOFTER

If balance is difficult, work each leg alternately. Gradually work up to doing both legs together. Reduce movement of hips and upper body, keeping hands on hips.

Roll Knees

1 Position feet close together and parallel.

2 Bend knees, place hands on legs above your knees and roll knees in circles. Keep your feet flat on the floor. Repeat 5 to 6 times each side.

Roll Hips

1 Bring hands to hips and roll hips slowly and smoothly. Repeat 5 to 6 times in each direction to loosen hips and release lower back.

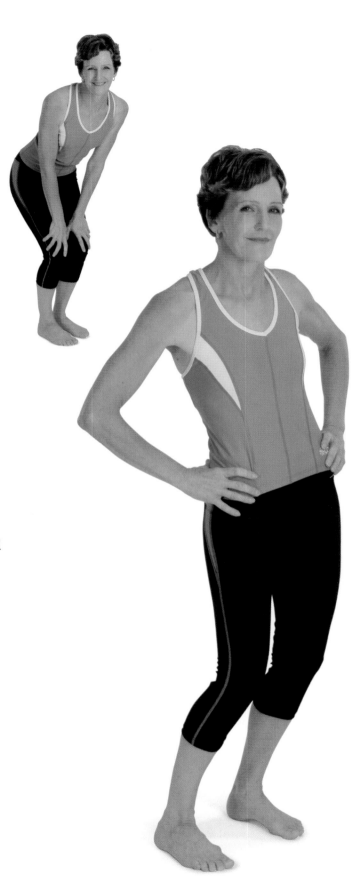

CIRCLE OF JOY

For further loosening and warming of
shoulders and upper body, and increasing
energy flow through your chest.

1 Stand in Tadasana, hands in Namaste
(prayer position – page 174).

2 Breathe in. Clasp hands as you breathe
out and push your palms away,
stretching arms forward with head
between your arms and folding forward
from your waist. Soften into your knees
if you need to.

3 Breathe in. Stretch arms overhead,
pressing clasped hands to the sky.
Breathe out. Release hands and arms
down behind your back.

4 Breathe in. Clasp hands and slowly
stretch arms back. Breathe out.
Bring arms straight forward palms
together. Breathe in. Hands back to
your heart. Repeat 3 times.

5 Hold in Namaste for 2 breaths,
eyes closed and observing effects.

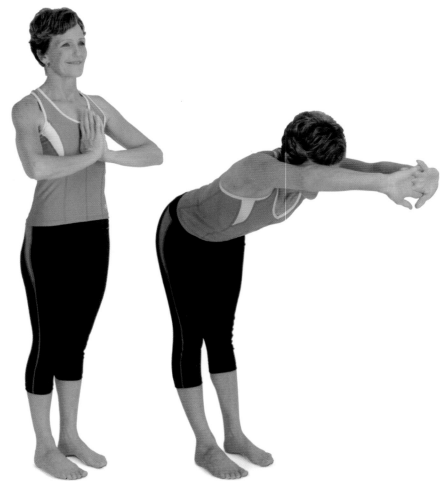

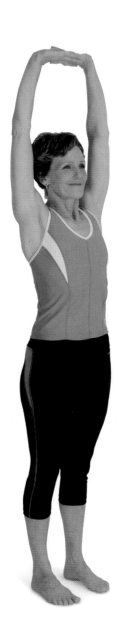
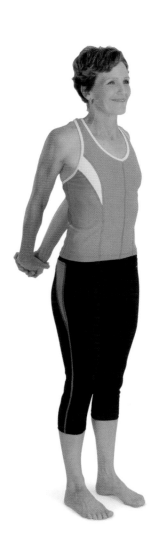
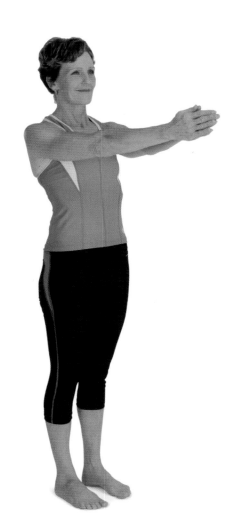

BEND & STRAIGHTEN LEGS

1 Position legs wide, feet in line and parallel. Bend one leg while stretching the other straight. Alternate from side-to-side.

2 Bend body forward slightly, placing hands and some weight on your bent leg. Keep foot on your straight leg side extended to the outer edge of that foot. Don't lock your knees. Repeat 6 times.

3 Stop movement. Bend knees and curl your body forward. Let head hang to release your neck. Bend elbows, wrap hands around elbows. Let breath flow.

4 Allow release and stretch through length of your back and neck. To come up, keep legs bent, sweep arms forward and up using your shoulders to lift.

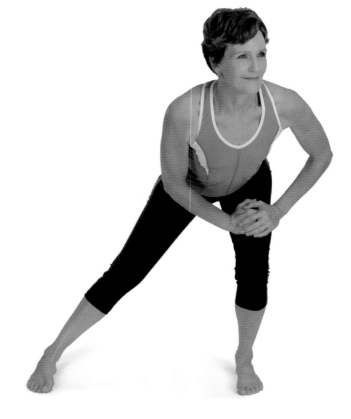

SOFTER

If you have blood pressure or heart problems, keep back level with the floor and head in line with, or higher than, your heart. Hands can support on your upper thighs.

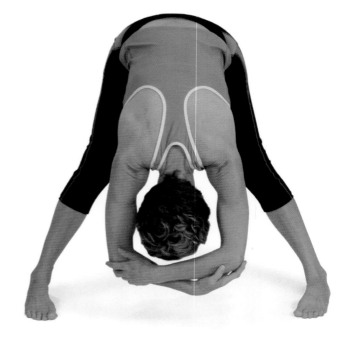

SUPPORTED SIDE STRETCH

1 Still with legs wide, extend arms to shoulder height. Breathe in. Breathe out. Tip arms to the left.

2 Rest left hand on your left leg extending right arm overhead and palm facing towards the floor.

3 Hold for 2 breaths. Return upright breathing in. Breathe out and repeat to the right.

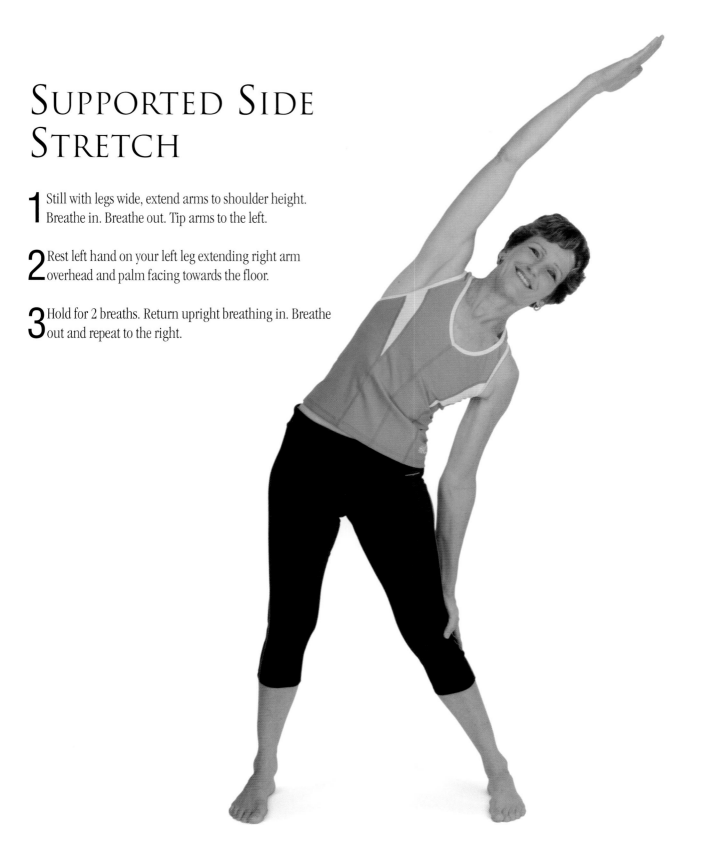

STANDING POSES

Loosen and relax your body between the postures if you are new to them. Repeat the Rotating Twist or Roll Hips, ensuring a release of any tension.

TRIANGLE POSE
TRIKONASANA

Benefits
- Strengthens all muscles and joints throughout your body
- Particularly strengthens legs, hips and lower back
- Lateral stretch for muscles supporting spine
- Awakens energy through your organs
- Attention to alignment keeps posture safe and allows freedom of energy flow

1 Position your feet at least 1.5 metres apart, in line and parallel. Lift left toes, swivel on heel and set toes out at 90 degrees to your body. Lift right heel back slightly, approximately 15 degrees. Front heel should be in line with the back instep. Try to keep your right hip back. Always attempt to keep your body in line with your legs.

2 Internally stretch tailbone towards the floor and feel a corresponding firming of your lower abdomen. This activates your pelvic core, providing stability and strength.

3 Stretch arms up level with shoulders. Breathe in. Extend from your heart to your fingertips. Breathe out. Fold from hip over your left leg.

4 Breathe in. Breathe out. Fold forward bringing left hand to the inside of your leg, opening your chest, stretching up with your right arm and both palms facing forward. Breathe evenly as you hold. Build up to holding for a few breaths.

5 Return your body upright on an inbreath. Lower arms and return feet to centre on an outbreath. Repeat on the other side.

CAUTION
Bend your front leg if you have back problems. If you have shoulder problems align them vertically and allow upper arm to rest behind your back.

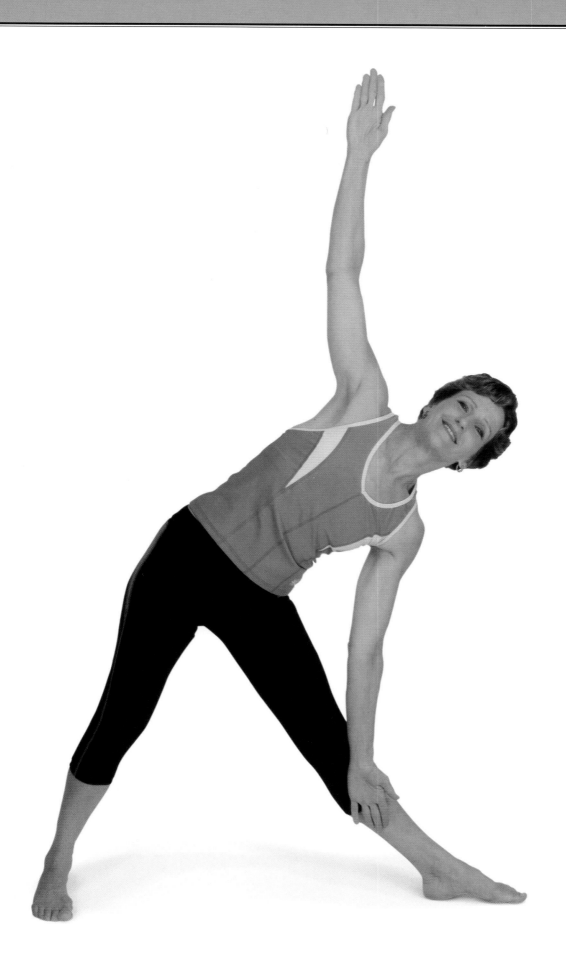

WARRIOR POSE
VIRABHADRASANA II

Benefits
- Strengthens legs, hips and lower back
- Stretches hip flexors (on the back leg)
- Strengthens quadricep muscles (on front leg, supporting the knee joint)
- Stimulates and tones kidneys and liver
- Fosters mental strength, endurance and confidence

1 Position your feet at least 1.5 metres apart, facing forward and parallel. Hands on hips. Lift left toes, swivel on heel and set toes out at 90 degrees. Lift right heel back to around 15 degrees. Activate your pelvic core as in Triangle Pose. Keep body upright, lifting through your heart.

2 Bend front leg into a lunge, adjusting distance between your feet if necessary. Front knee should be directly above your ankle and in line with your toes. Back leg should be straight and strong with pressure on the outer edge of your back foot. If back leg feels weak, shorten the distance between your feet and reduce the depth of the lunge in your front leg.

3 Raise arms level with your shoulders, keeping a straight line from fingertip to fingertip, palms facing the floor. Look forward over your front hand. Breathe as you hold. Build up to holding for a few breaths.

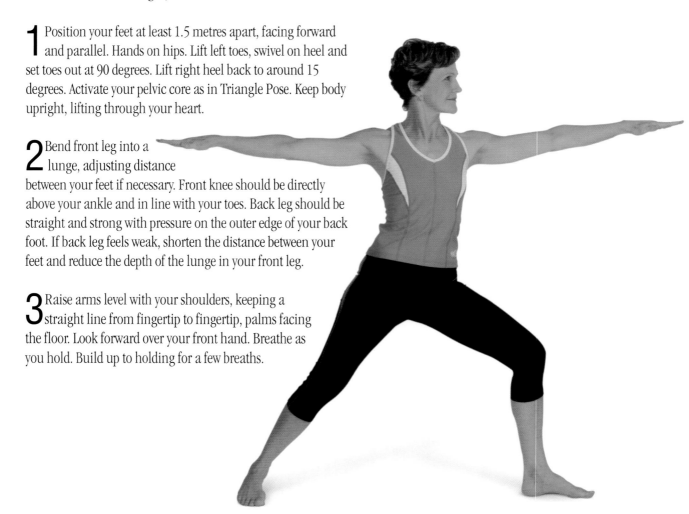

ARCHER POSE

1 From Warrior Pose, breathe out and tip back.

2 Bring right hand to rest on your right leg. Breathe in. Stretch left arm forward and up in a straight diagonal line. Hold for 1 or 2 breathes, then return to Warrior Pose.

3 Lower hands to your hips, straighten front leg and turn feet to the front.

4 Repeat Warrior and Archer Poses on the other side.

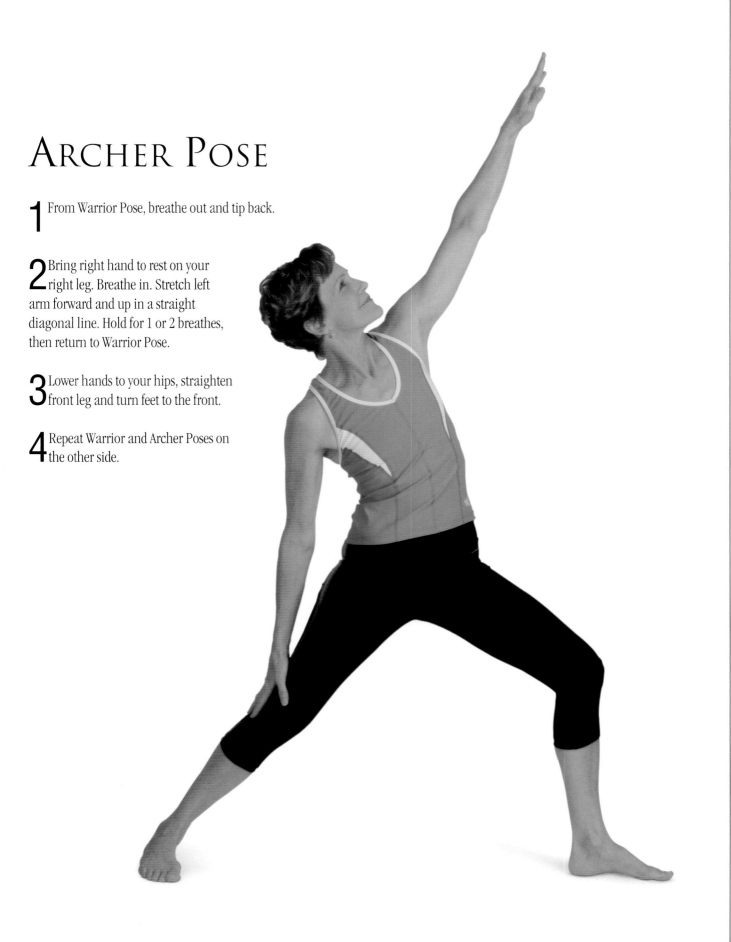

INTENSE FORWARD STRETCH (Bliss Fix)
Prasarita Padottanasana

Benefits
- Forward stretch relaxes your back and elongates your spine
- Calms your mind
- Soothes your nervous system
- This version has a stimulating effect on your lymph glands (and other glands), boosts your immune system and ensures production of 'happy hormones'

1 Position your feet at least 1.5 metres apart, facing forward and parallel.

2 Breathe in. Raise arms to shoulder height. Breathe out. Fold from your hips taking your body forward and down.

3 Clasp hands behind your back. Slowly straighten arms back and up taking hands towards the ceiling. Keep your neck relaxed and shoulders away from your ears.

4 To come out of the pose, bend your knees in a semi-squat, thighs strong. Take arms out wide, level with your shoulders. Lift with your shoulders to come up. Roll hips to ensure your body feels at ease.

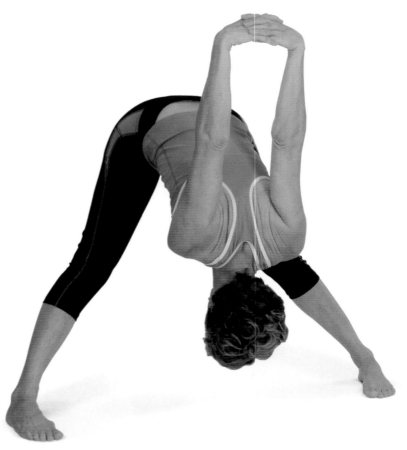

SOFTER

Bend your knees. Keep arms relaxed on your back. Or, bend your knees and bring hands on to your legs for support, raising back level with the floor and straightening your arms.

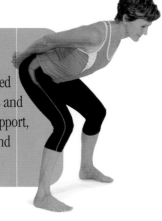

BALANCE

With all balances, find a spot in front of you where you can fix a soft gaze, helping your mind to focus.

TREE POSE
VRKSASANA

Benefits
- Provides valuable weight bearing to increase bone mass
- Strengthens muscles and joints
- Improves posture and alignment
- Improves mental focus and concentration

1 Ground firmly through your right foot, gradually taking weight off your left foot. Using your right hand to help, bring your left foot up onto your right leg, foot facing straight down. Aim to bring left heel into your right groin. Employ basic alignments as in Tadasana (page 142), pressing your right leg against your raised foot.

2 When foundation is strong, stretch your arms up overhead, palms together. Aim towards bringing elbows straight, arms a little behind your ears. Hold while breathing deeply and smoothly. Connect your consciousness with the trees – the lungs of the earth.

3 Return hands to prayer position at your heart. Slowly release your left leg. Repeat on the other side. Roll hips to ease hips and lower back.

SOFTER
Stand with back supported against a wall. Only take your raised foot as high as your body allows.

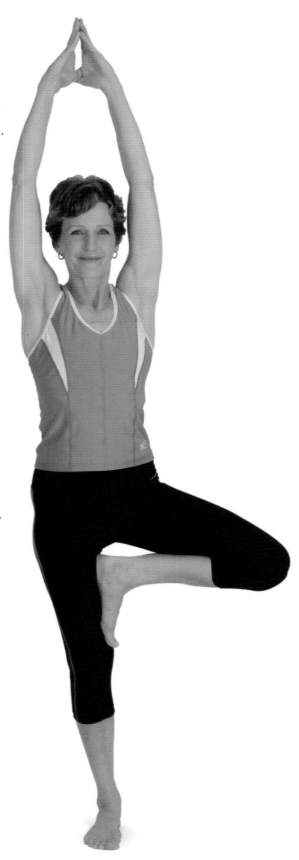

FLOOR POSES

CAT POSE
MARJARASANA

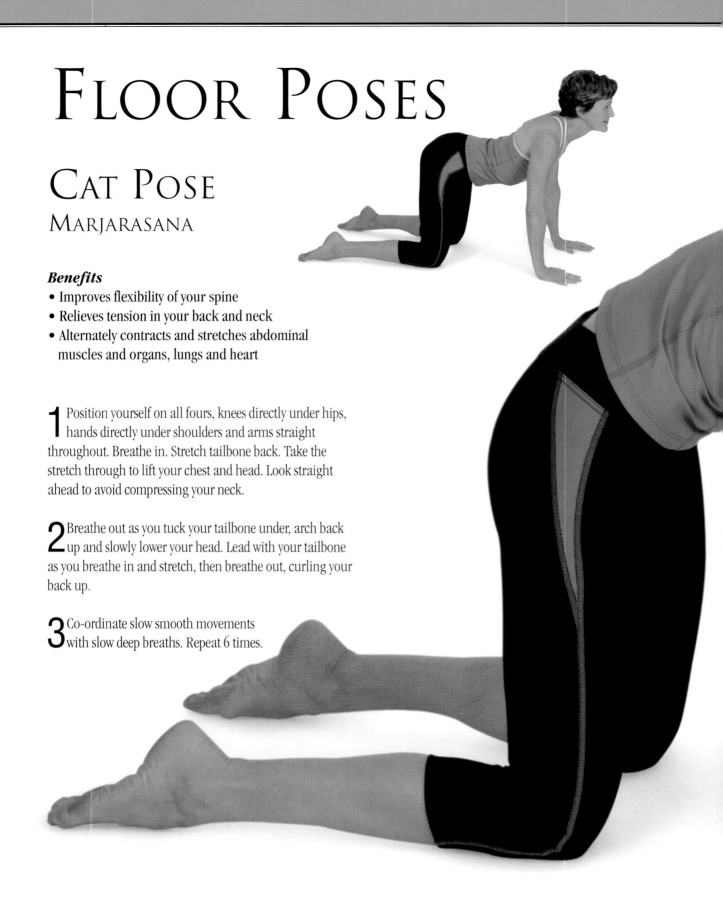

Benefits
- Improves flexibility of your spine
- Relieves tension in your back and neck
- Alternately contracts and stretches abdominal muscles and organs, lungs and heart

1 Position yourself on all fours, knees directly under hips, hands directly under shoulders and arms straight throughout. Breathe in. Stretch tailbone back. Take the stretch through to lift your chest and head. Look straight ahead to avoid compressing your neck.

2 Breathe out as you tuck your tailbone under, arch back up and slowly lower your head. Lead with your tailbone as you breathe in and stretch, then breathe out, curling your back up.

3 Co-ordinate slow smooth movements with slow deep breaths. Repeat 6 times.

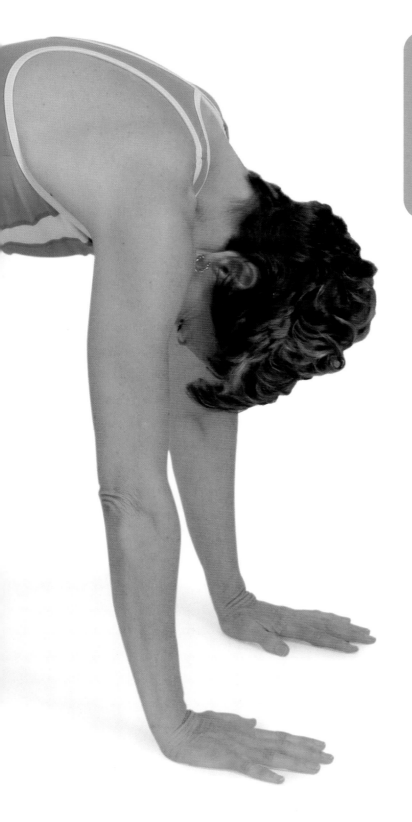

VARIATION

For a deeper stretch into your lower back.

The inbreath is the same. The outbreath is in
3 parts – tailbone under, bend elbows to the
floor, take hips back to your heels.
Repeat 3 times.

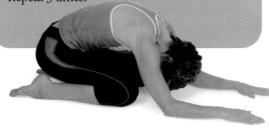

DOG POSE

SVANASANA

Benefits

- Strengthens all muscles and joints, particularly arms, shoulders and upper body
- Relieves arthritis and fatigue
- It is a part inversion (when you partly turn upside down) with the same rejuvenating benefits to your brain
- Lengthens and strengthens your spine
- Aids organ function and breathing

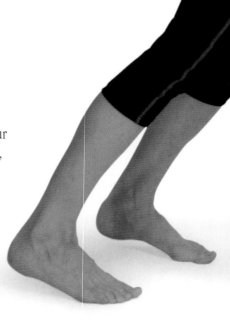

1 Sit back on heels, feet up on toes. Extend your arms forward, shoulder width apart. Try to align middle fingers with the outer edge of your shoulders. Spread fingers and plant hands firmly on the floor, particularly pressing down on the balls of your fingers so your wrists aren't doing all the work.

2 Press into your toes, moving your hips up and back, stretching your tailbone up. Don't straighten your legs right away if the backs of your legs are tight.

3 Keep neck soft and your head between your arms, looking straight through to your legs. Draw shoulders away from your ears, broaden and flatten across upper back, directing your chest towards your thighs. Avoid dipping into your lower back.

4 If legs allow, slowly straighten directing your heels back towards the floor. Focus on the action through your back first before attending to your legs.

SOFTER

Keep knees bent. Alternately bend and straighten legs to encourage hamstring muscles to stretch. For weak wrists, roll a towel into a sausage shape and grip your hands over this roll.

3-Legged Dog
For a Challenge

1 Bring feet close together and raise right leg off the floor. Diagonally line up your arms, back and raised leg. Hold for 2 breaths.

2 Return leg to the floor and repeat with your left leg.

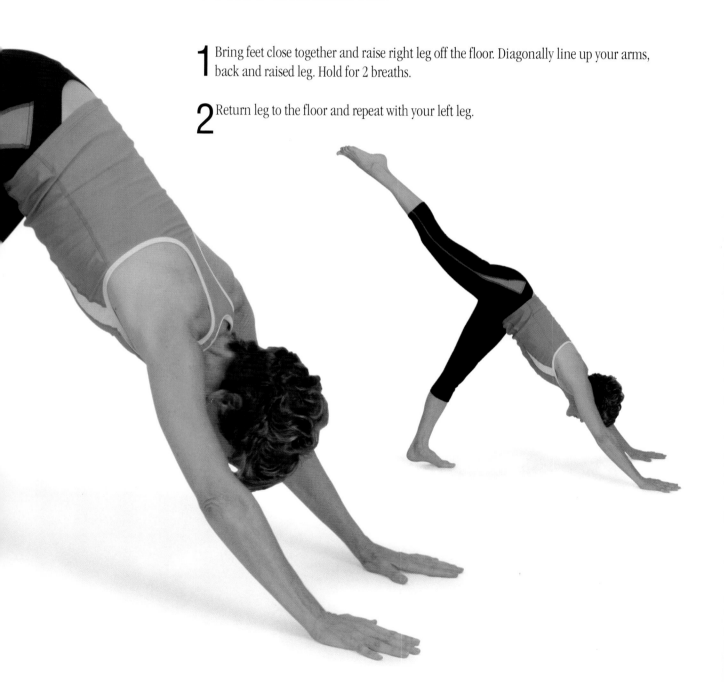

CHILD POSE
PRANATASANA

1 Kneel back with buttocks on heels, body resting on thighs, arms alongside your body and forehead resting on the floor. Hold for 1 to 2 minutes.

Improvise with one or more of the following if this is not giving a feeling of ease and release:
• Make a space between your knees to fit your body
• Place a folded blanket or towel between your thighs and calves
• Place a cushion or folded blanket under your forehead
• Bring arms forward, make fists one on top of the other and rest forehead on your fists

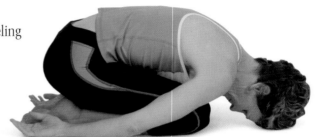

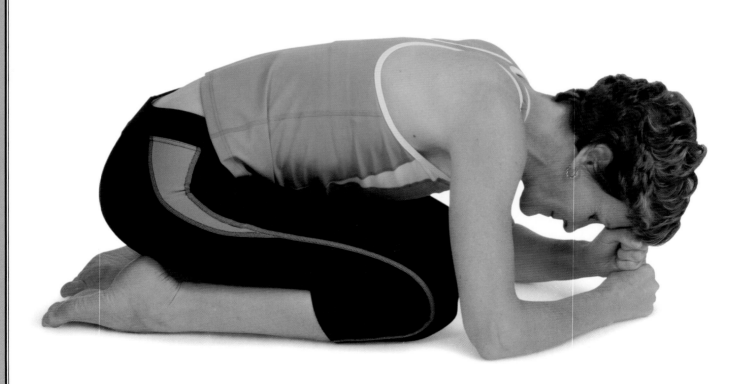

PRONE POSES

Slide forward to lie on your stomach.

BACK BENDS

Benefits
- Stimulates and tones kidneys and adrenal glands
- Maintains strength and suppleness of spine and supporting muscles
- Stretches and tones organs and muscles at the front of your body

CAUTION
Seek advice from your medical practitioner if you have any spinal conditions and/or injuries. Not suitable during pregnancy or if you have a hernia.

SPHINX POSE

1 Stretch arms forward and legs behind.

2 Walk hands back until elbows are under your shoulders, forearms facing forward, upper body gently lifted off the floor.

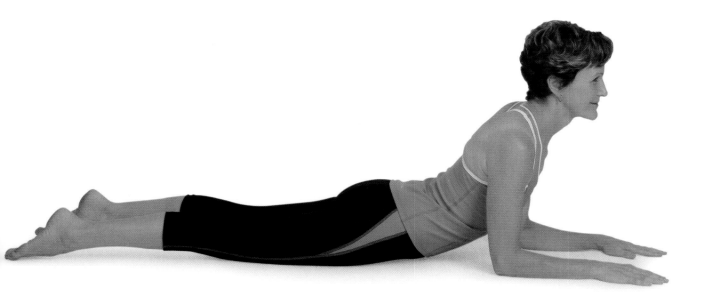

COBRA POSE

BHUJANGASANA

1 Bring hands under your shoulders, elbows tucked back towards your ribs. Keep thighs actively pressed against the floor, gently stretching back into your feet. Avoid hunching your shoulders.

2 Press hands into the floor and lift upper body from the floor leading with your chest and keeping head in line with your spine. Build up to holding for 3 or more breaths.

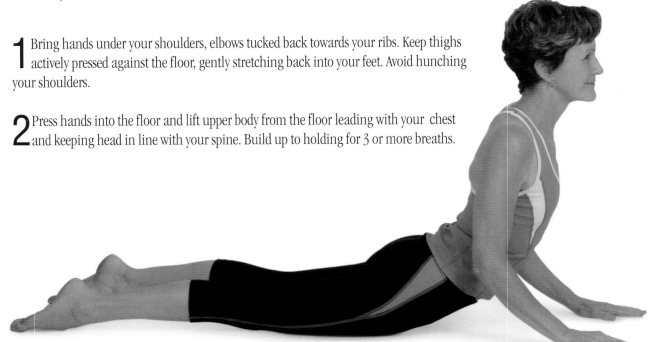

CROCODILE POSE

1 To rest, lower body to floor. Bend elbows, placing forearms in front and resting forehead on your arms.

2 Rock hips a little from side-to-side to release any tension in your back. Then lie still and observe your breath.

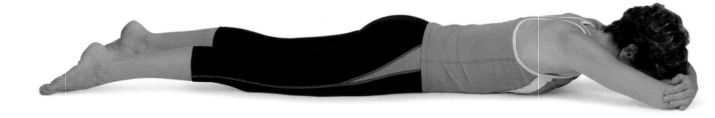

RECLINING POSES

Benefits
- Stabilises your back and hips after the other postures
- Prepares body and mind for inversions and relaxation

ROLL ON THE BACK

1 Clasp hands around bent knees and circle your knees slowly a few times in each direction.

2 Make as wide a circle as you can in order to massage a large area of your back. This also calms your mind and nervous system.

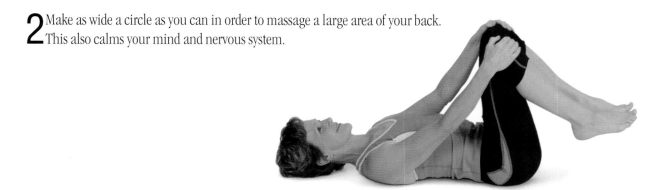

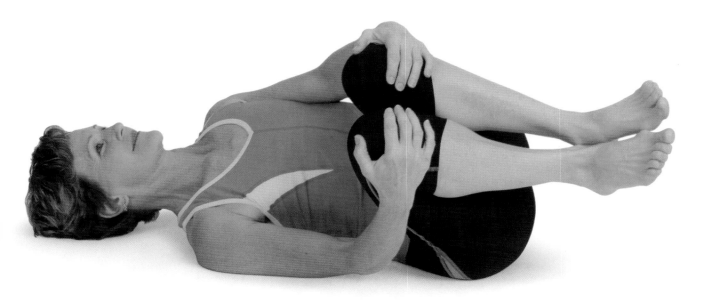

AIRWALK

Benefits

- Strengthens abdominal muscles, particularly your transverse abdominus, while keeping your back safe on the floor
- Using alternate limbs gives a cross-patterning effect on your brain, providing stimulation

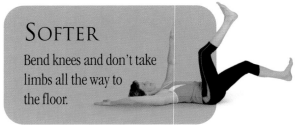

SOFTER
Bend knees and don't take limbs all the way to the floor.

1 Stretch your arms and legs up taking hands and feet towards the ceiling.

2 Lower left leg down to the floor while taking right arm back to the floor behind. Return them both back upright as you simultaneously lower your right leg down and your left arm back behind.

3 Keep the movement going smoothly and with an even breath. Only briefly touch the floor before returning. If you rest, it takes more strength to lift your limbs back up.

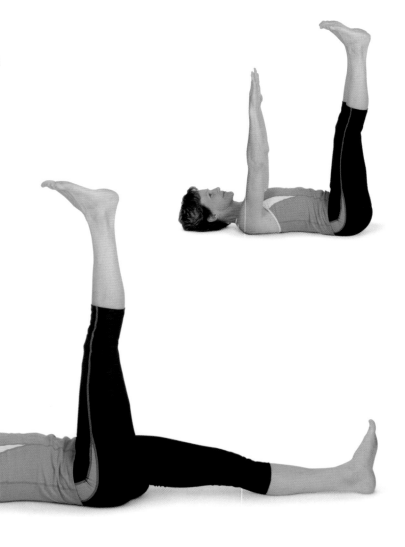

HANDS AROUND KNEES
APANASANA

1 Clasp hands around your knees and rest. Allow knees to press lightly into your arms, keeping your abdominals free, allowing the area to soften with your breath.

SWAYING TWIST

Benefits
• Keeps spine and supporting muscles aligned, toned and supple
• Stretches muscles and organs in front of your body

2 Release hands, straightening arms up and taking hands towards the ceiling. Knees are bent with feet off the floor. Breathe out. Take legs across to the left and let your arms lower across to the right. Breathe in. Return to the centre.

3 Breathe out. Take legs across to the right and let arms lower across to the left. Keep the swaying movement going slowly and smoothly, co-ordinating your breath.

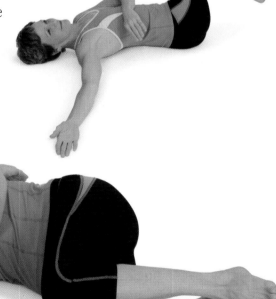

SOFTER
Keep arms on the floor out level with your shoulders.

FLOATING BRIDGE

Benefits

- Strengthens thighs, buttocks, pelvic floor and abdominals
- Aligns spine, particularly your sacrum and lower back
- Increases flexibility throughout
- The arm movements stretch and release shoulders and upper back

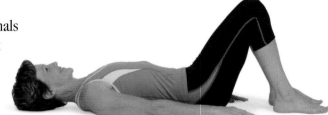

1 Position your feet close to buttocks and hip width apart. Keep feet and knees hip width apart and parallel throughout. Arms alongside your body.

2 On an inbreath, slowly roll your hips off the floor continuing through the length of your back until you have a diagonal line from shoulders up to your knees. At the same time raise your arms up overhead.

3 As you breathe out, slowly roll your back down to the floor returning your arms alongside your body. Synchronise breath and movement. Press feet firmly into the floor to access the strength of your legs.

4 Aim to roll your back, separating your vertebrae, rather than moving it as a single unit. Try 3 to 4 times and build up to 6 times.

SOFTER

Keep arms on the floor beside your body, or take arms out wide level with your shoulders.

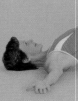

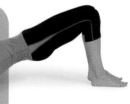

LEGS UP THE WALL

1 Sit with your body at right angles to a wall. Lean back on your hands and swing your body and legs around, lying down with your legs up the wall and buttocks as close as possible to the wall. Arms rest comfortably at your sides. Stay in position for 3 to 5 minutes.

2 Or, going a little further, bend your knees, pressing feet into the wall and lift buttocks off the floor. Slide bolster or stacked blankets under your sacrum for support. Rest here 3 to 5 minutes. Reverse the process slowly to come down. Once removing the support, lower your back down to the floor.

To return from either version, bend your knees towards your chest. Roll over to the right side and rest briefly before stretching out on the floor for the next pose.

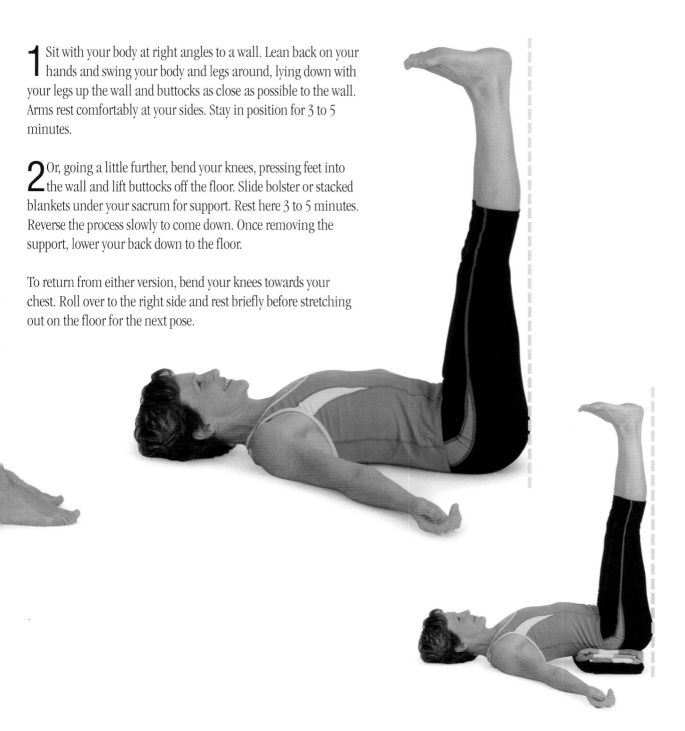

HALF SHOULDERSTAND

Benefits

- Stimulates and tones all your glands, improving hormone function and overall health, wellbeing and immunity
- Reverses the pull of gravity on joints, muscles, organs and circulation – hence its rejuvenating effects
- Relieves fatigue, hemorrhoids, prolapse and varicose veins
- Refreshes your mind and nervous system, providing a sense of clarity
- Strengthens your back and abdominals

1 Once your legs are up, ensure that there is pressure on the centre of the back of your head, NOT on the length of your neck. Your neck remains in its natural curve, chin lower than your forehead and a triangular line of support from the centre of the back of your head along your upper arms to your elbows.

2 Roll back and forth on the floor a few times, taking your legs back overhead until you feel comfortable. Wriggle your shoulder blades closer together, bringing your elbows in close under your body.

3 Raise your legs up, feet above your hips, while lowering your hips onto your hands. If your elbows are not brought in close enough, the weight bearing won't be correct so come down carefully and do Legs Up The Wall. Hold for a few breaths and relax. Try to build up to holding 1 to 3 minutes.

4 To come down, bend knees towards your chest and slowly roll your back down to the floor, keeping hands on your back for support.

CAUTION

This is a safe inversion when done correctly. However, if you have any neck or back problems, eye problems such as detached retina, high blood pressure, heart problems or if menstruating or pregnant, do the softer version (Legs Up The Wall).

Corpse Pose

Savasana

Provides complete withdrawal of the senses, relaxing your body and mind while keeping clarity and awareness.

1 Lie on your back, lift head and look to your feet ensuring your head and spine are aligned. Allow your back and neck to settle into their natural curves. Take your legs a little apart so feet can flop, relaxing ankles, knees and hips.

2 Take arms a little away from your body, palms facing up and fingers lightly curled. Shoulders are broad and relaxed.

3 If there is any discomfort in your lower back, place a support (folded blanket or pillow) under your knees. If there is any discomfort in your neck, place a small support under the back of your head. Keep chin low towards your chest.

4 Slowly scan through your body, breathing into and relaxing each part of your body. Then merge with your breath and simply be.

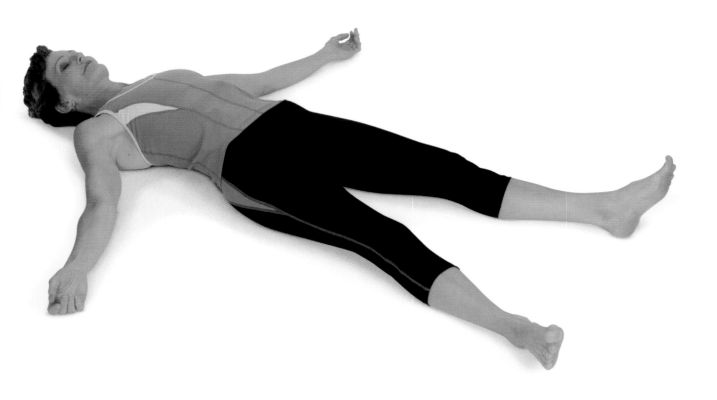

MEDITATION

Benefits
- Lowers stress levels
- Boosts your body's immune system
- Potential to heal physically, emotionally and mentally
- Calms your mind, giving better clarity, focus and efficiency
- Ability to respond consciously to life's situations rather than reacting from old habits

Due to the ever-changing condition of our work-a-day mind, the meditation experience can alter from day-to-day. Therefore regular practice is the key, and over time we find that our so-called 'monkey mind' becomes more disciplined – at times entering into relative quietness – which enables access to the deeper levels of the mind, levels where we connect with our intuition, creativity and inspiration.

When beginning to practise aim for the same time each day, in a place where you feel relaxed and won't be disturbed. It is preferable to meditate for 5 to 10 minutes daily than for longer periods less often. Meditation is about doing less and 'being' more and retaining awareness in the present moment.

Meditation is the spontaneous progression from concentration to that one-pointed focus where subject and object merge. Your mind is alert but relaxed and open to that blissful state of union with 'all that there is' (Samadhi).

1 Find an object of concentration that suits you personally:
- Watching your breath
- Visualising an image – a beautiful scene, a single object, a spiritual person
- Listening to calming music
- Mentally reciting a mantra

2 As your mind throws thoughts up to the surface of your consciousness, gently bring it back to the object of concentration. It is not about completely blanking your mind but more about letting thoughts flow by without giving them attention. It is like becoming a witness – detaching from the external world, watching but not participating. It does get easier with practise and the benefits are priceless.

3 Sit cross-legged, back straight with shoulders, face and jaw relaxed. Place hands gently in your lap. You may create a mudra (gesture or seal) with your hands to enhance the energy of centredness by joining thumb and index fingertips in a circle, extending your remaining fingers and placing backs of hands on your knees.

4 Close your eyes, relax and focus on the object of concentration.

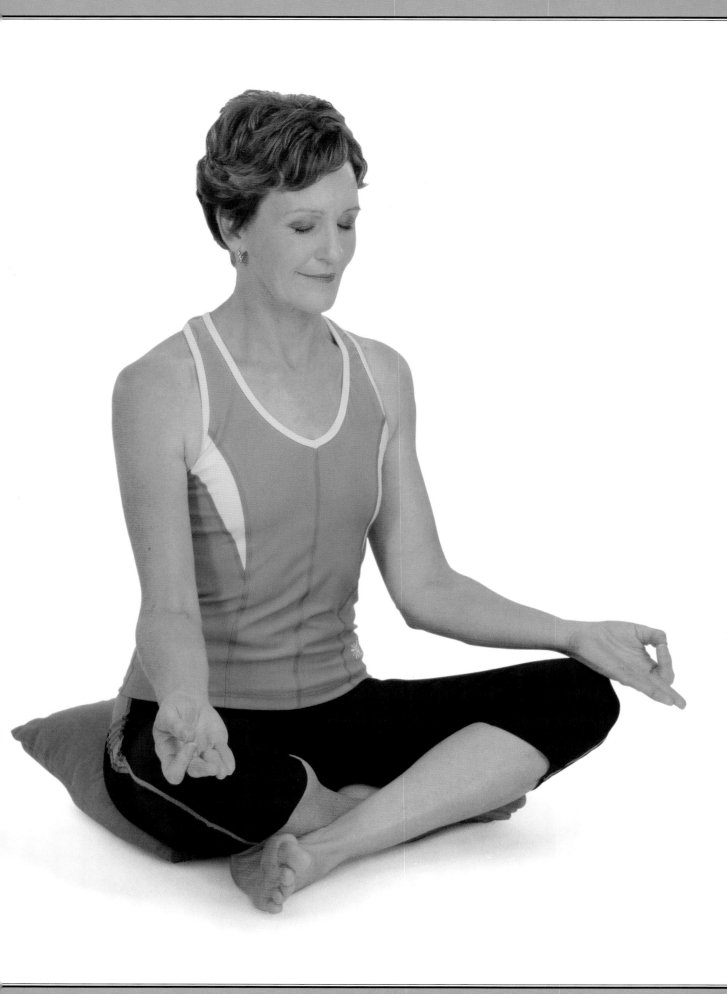

PARTNER-SHARING YOGA
INTRODUCTION

Partner work can bring an added dimension to the yoga postures. Using the support and assistance of a partner, it is easier to relax and deepen into the stretches. For that very reason, it is important to keep focused and aware in order not to go beyond the limits your body may have at this present time.

Sharing postures with a partner opens your awareness to include another person, adding to the enjoyment and sense of achievement that yoga postures can give. It is ideal to find a partner who is roughly the same height and build and who has similar ability as yourself. However, I have chosen postures where these requirements are not essential. Keep the channels of communication open. Give your partner constant feedback as to how far you want to go and when you are ready to release out of a pose.

If you wish to expand your partner work or have any doubts whatsoever, consult a qualified yoga teacher.

CAUTION

Take the usual care that you would when practising alone. With any back or joint injuries consult a medical practitioner first and seek guidance from a qualified yoga teacher.

NAMASTE

(A traditional greeting meaning 'the divinity within me greets the divinity within you')

1 Stand facing your partner with hands in prayer position at your heart centre.

2 Look into each other's eyes and make a connection, silently dedicating this practice to the highest benefit of all.

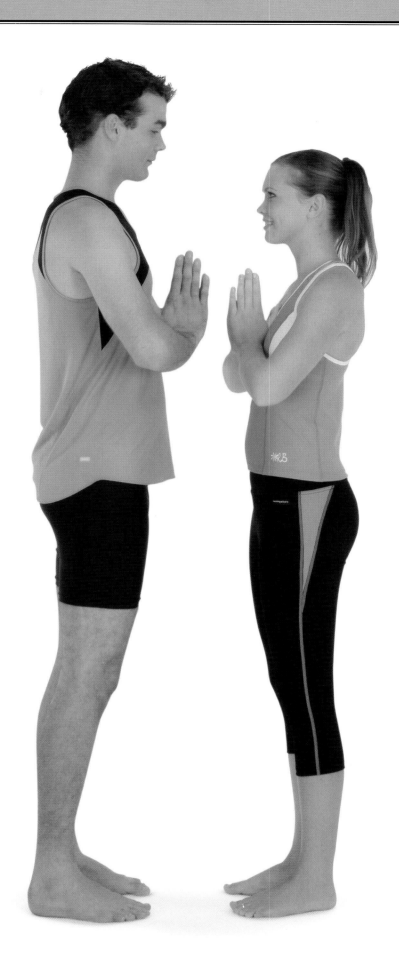

PARTNER-SHARING YOGA *(continued)*

BACK-TO-BACK SIDE STRETCH

It's a nice warm-up, loosening shoulders and upper back and gently stretching hips, back and side muscles.

1 Standing back-to-back either hold hands or entwine hands around each other's wrists. Try to synchronise your breath.

2 Breath in. Stretch up one pair of arms and on an outbreath, continue moving over to the side keeping the upstretched arms overhead. Keep hips level and upper shoulders back.

3 Hold for a breath or two. Return upright on an inbreath, lowering arms to sides on an outbreath. When ready, repeat on the other side.

4 If you prefer, you could start up a swaying movement, slowly and smoothly taking arms up, over to one side, back upright and down to starting position, alternating sides.

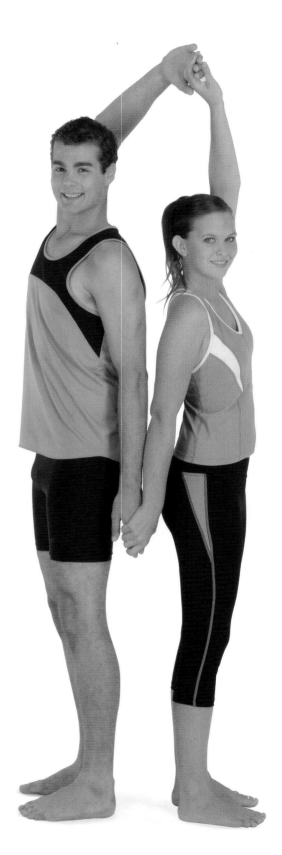

SUSPENSION BRIDGE

1 Facing each other take hold of your partner's wrists in a monkey grip.

2 Step back until you can fold forward, hinging from your hips and bringing your backs parallel to the floor, a right angle at your hips and your arms straight. Stretch back into your tailbone breathing evenly, keeping your head in line with your spine. Your partner's weight assists your stretch.

3 Broaden across your shoulders opening your chest towards the floor. Try not to hunch your shoulders around your ears. Take time to relax into the stretch.

4 To come out, bend knees slightly and walk towards each other as you come upright.

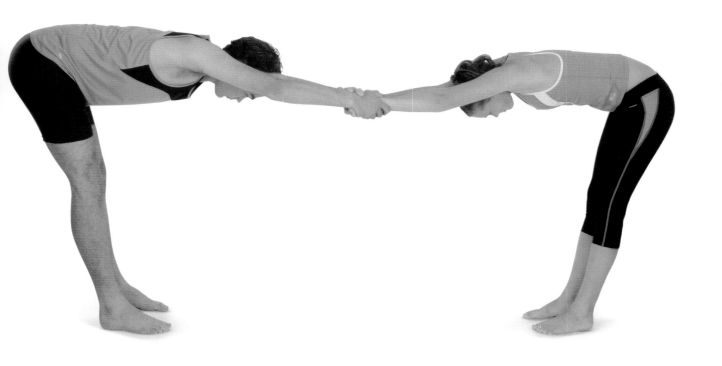

LEAN BACK

1 Still facing each other with a monkey grip around each other's wrists, come close enough so that your toes are touching. (You may have to adjust this distance according to the length of your arms.) Slowly lean back, straightening into your arms, keeping your bodies straight, shoulders low and tucking your buttocks under.

2 Take time to trust your partner's weight supporting you as you lean back. If, and when, you feel comfortable with your partner's support you could tuck your buttocks in further and arch your back into a backbend.

3 When ready to return, bend your arms bringing elbows back to your body enabling your partner to return upright.

Remember to keep communicating with your partner and indicate if the stretch is too strong and needs to be adjusted, and when you are ready to come out of a pose. Always move slowly with consideration for your partner as well as awareness of your own body.

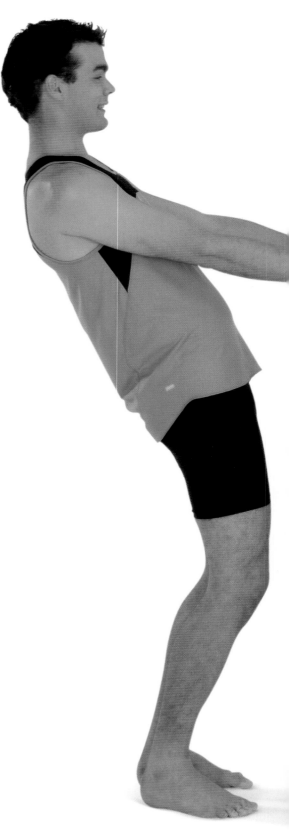

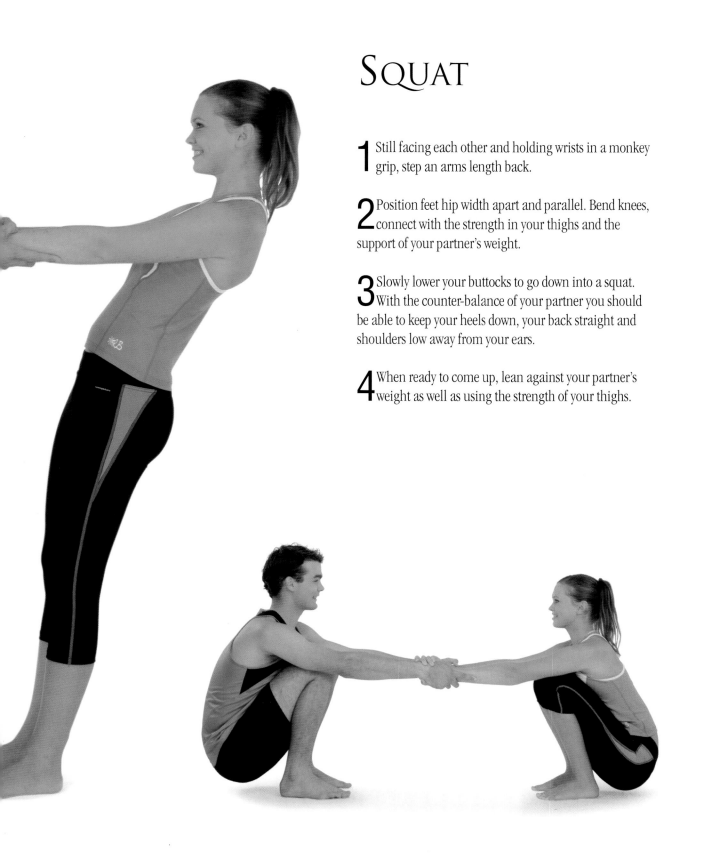

Squat

1 Still facing each other and holding wrists in a monkey grip, step an arms length back.

2 Position feet hip width apart and parallel. Bend knees, connect with the strength in your thighs and the support of your partner's weight.

3 Slowly lower your buttocks to go down into a squat. With the counter-balance of your partner you should be able to keep your heels down, your back straight and shoulders low away from your ears.

4 When ready to come up, lean against your partner's weight as well as using the strength of your thighs.

WARRIOR POSE
VIRABHADRASANA II

Here you will be able to compare how this posture feels with the assistance of a partner after trying it solo in the general class.

1 Face in the opposite direction to your partner and bring the outer edges of your closest feet together. Take hold of your partner's wrist closest to you.

2 Step each of your outer legs into a lunge, making sure that your knee is aligned directly over your ankle and in line with your toes.

3 Keep bodies in line with your legs and extend your outer arms forward at shoulder height. Your partner's weight assists you in staying upright and strong in the pose, making you more aware of the strength in your back leg.

4 To come out, straighten your bent leg, lower arms, turn to the centre and walk your feet together. Repeat the pose on the other side.

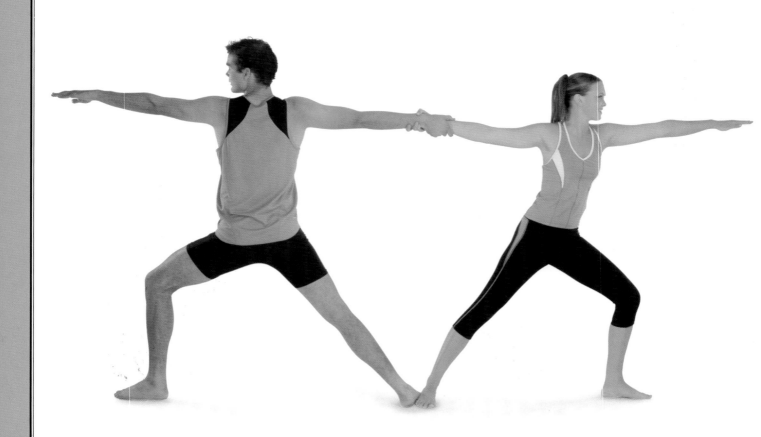

HERO POSE
VIRABHADRASANA I

1 Stand facing each other, step your right foot forward and connect the inner edge of your foot with that of your partner. Step back with your left foot and go into a lunge with your right leg.

2 Keep your hips facing forward and your back leg straight and strong. Don't roll on to the instep of your back foot. If there is any strain to your knee or foot, raise your heel off the floor. Shorten the distance between your feet if you can't keep your back leg strong.

3 Raise arms forward to chest height and press palms against your partner's palms. Try to keep your arms straight and shoulders low. This brings awareness to your upper body, opens your chest and strengthens your upper back. It also helps to balance and stabilise your legs and hips.

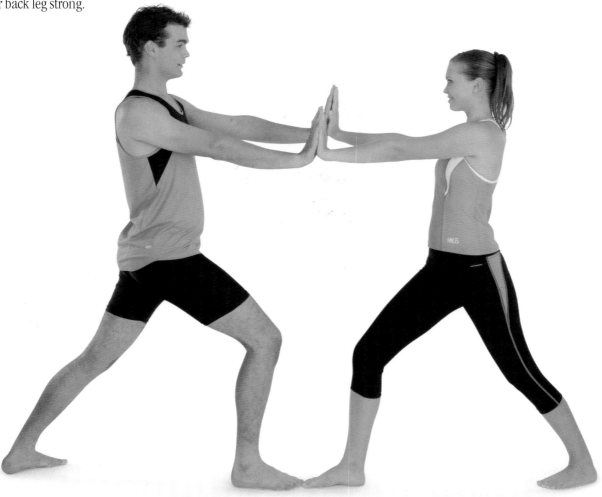

SIDE STRETCH
DOUBLE MOON

1 Stand side-by-side about half a metre apart. Hold hands. Breathe in. Stretch your outer arms overhead. Breathe out. Stretch sideways towards each other, bringing your upper hands/fingers to touch.

2 Keep your hips facing forward and upper shoulders back. Hold briefly breathing evenly.

3 Return arms upright on an inbreath, lowering arms to sides on an outbreath. Change sides and repeat.

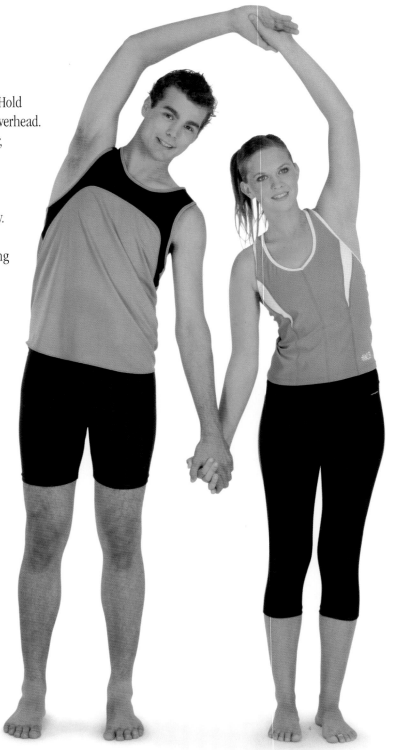

TREE POSE
VRKSASANA

1 Stand closely, side-by-side. Slowly raise your outer foot, using a hand to help if needed. Place your foot against your standing leg and follow directions as described earlier (page 157).

2 Raise your inner arm up overhead and hold your partner's hand (or arm depending on discrepancy in lengths).

3 Raise your outer hand and join with your partner's at heart level in prayer position. After a few breaths, release and change sides.

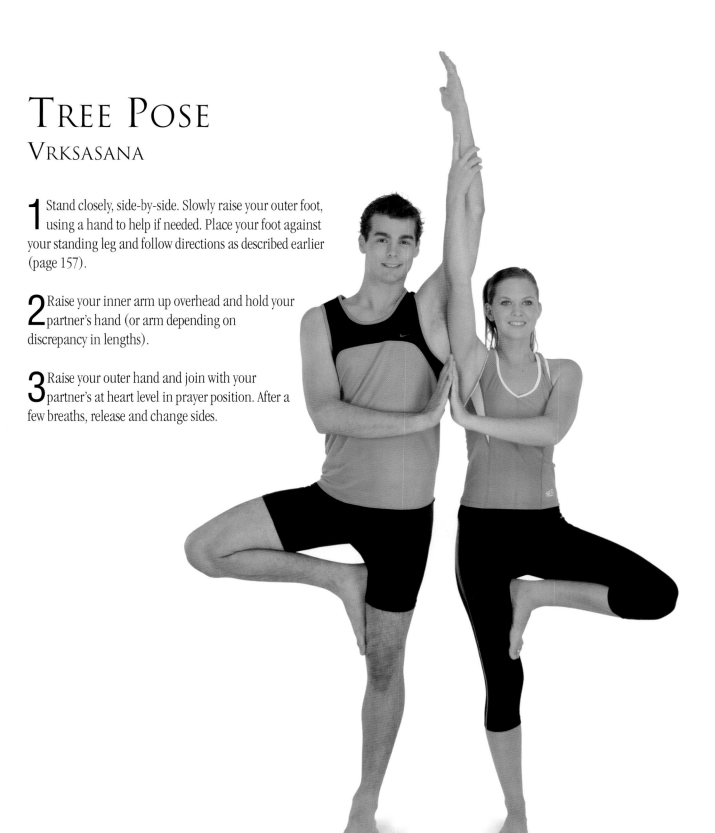

DOG POSE

SVANASANA

The next three poses are partner-assisted – one performing the posture (**A**) and the other assisting (**B**). **A** performs all three first before changing roles.

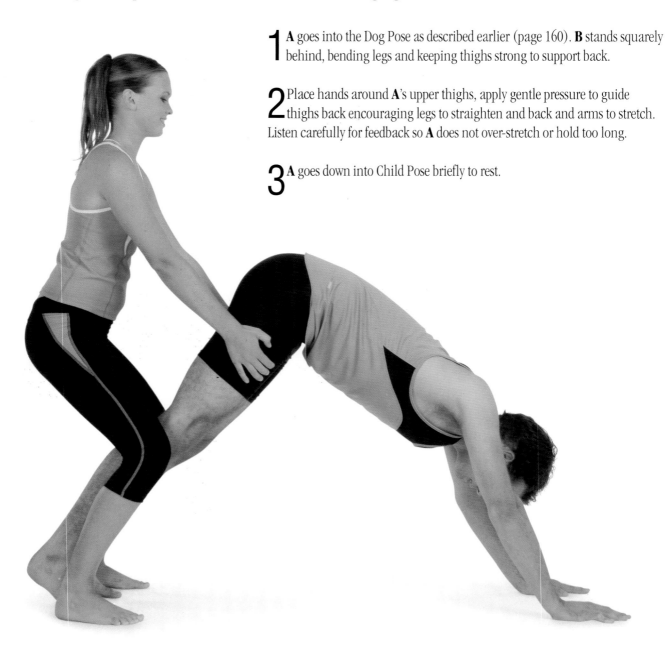

1 **A** goes into the Dog Pose as described earlier (page 160). **B** stands squarely behind, bending legs and keeping thighs strong to support back.

2 Place hands around **A**'s upper thighs, apply gentle pressure to guide thighs back encouraging legs to straighten and back and arms to stretch. Listen carefully for feedback so **A** does not over-stretch or hold too long.

3 **A** goes down into Child Pose briefly to rest.

COBRA POSE
BHUJANGASANA

1 **A** lies prone on the floor arms alongside their body. **B** stands over **A**, feet each side of **A**'s thighs. Note: It is important for **B** to bend their knees and use the strength of their thighs (not the back) for lifting.

2 Grip each other's wrists. On an exhalation from **A**, **B** slowly and smoothly lifts **A**'s upper body from the floor. **A** uses no effort and indicates when they'd like to be lowered back to the floor.

3 If **A** wishes to try Cobra Pose alone (page 164) there could be a pleasant surprise – more lift and ease. **A** then goes into Child Pose.

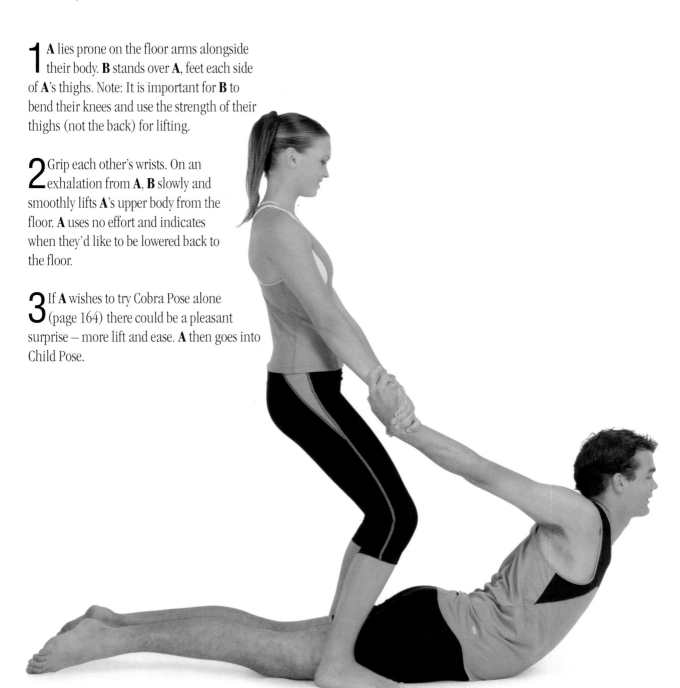

Partner-Sharing Yoga *(continued)*

Child Pose
Pranatasana

1 **B** kneels alongside **A** and places one hand on their lower back, the other on their upper back.

2 With gentle pressure imagine you are lengthening **A**'s back, lower hand moving towards their tailbone and the upper hand towards their head. You don't have to be heavy-handed to give **A**'s back a nice release and stretch.

Change roles and repeat the last three postures.

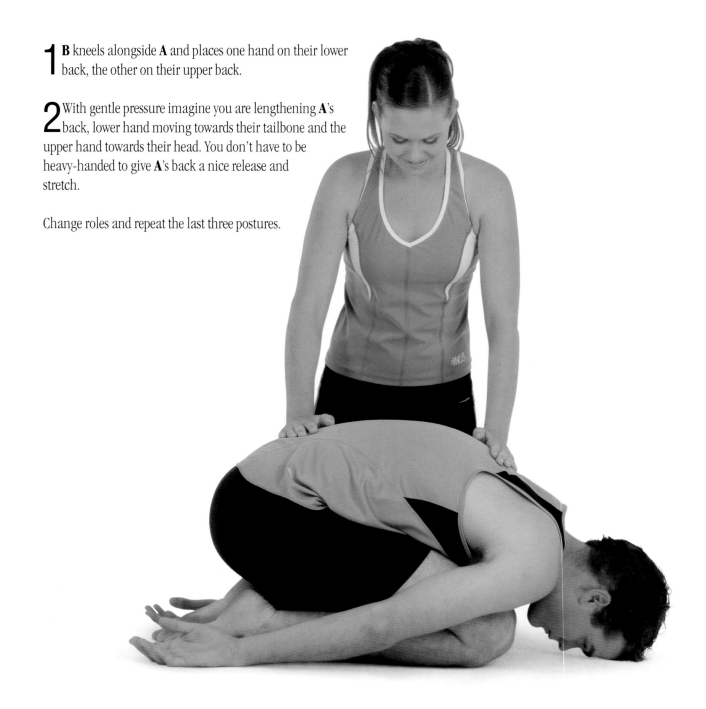

SEATED BACK-TO-BACK

1 Either cross-legged or with legs stretched straight in front, lean straight backs against each other.

2 Take a couple of minutes to be aware of your breathing – the slow rhythm. Then bring your awareness to your partner's breath. Maybe your breathing will synchronise, flowing in unison.

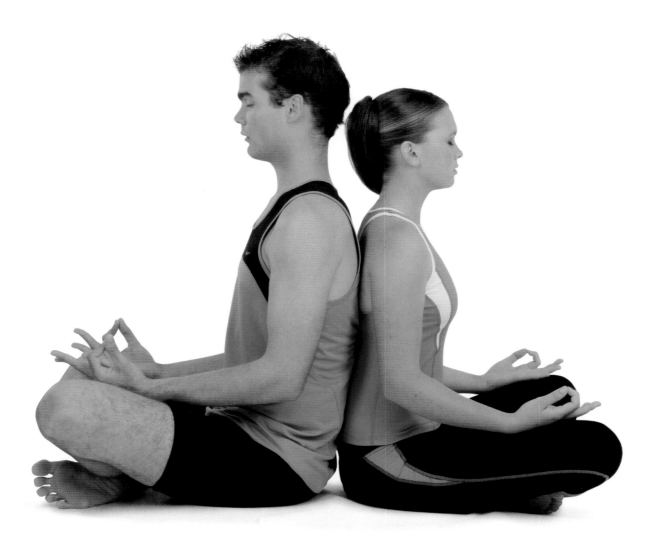

BACK-TO-BACK TWIST

1 Cross legs, take your right hand to your own left knee and your left hand to your partner's right knee.

2 Keep backs connected, twist gently and look over your left shoulder. Hold for a few breaths. Release slowly back to centre and repeat to the opposite side.

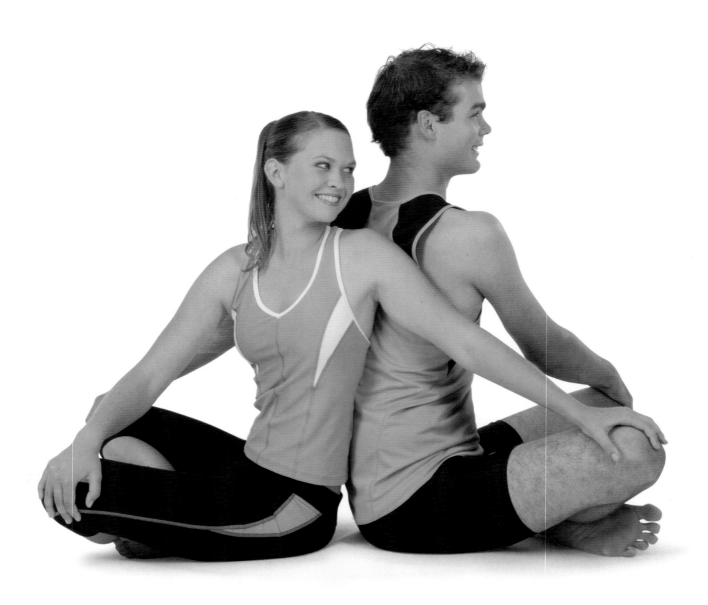

SIDE STRETCH

1 Place hands together at each side. On an inbreath stretch up one pair of arms. On an outbreath stretch over to the opposite side. Hands on the floor provide support.

2 Keep both pairs of buttocks on the floor and backs connected.

3 Return arms upright breathing in, and back to the floor breathing out. Repeat on the other side.

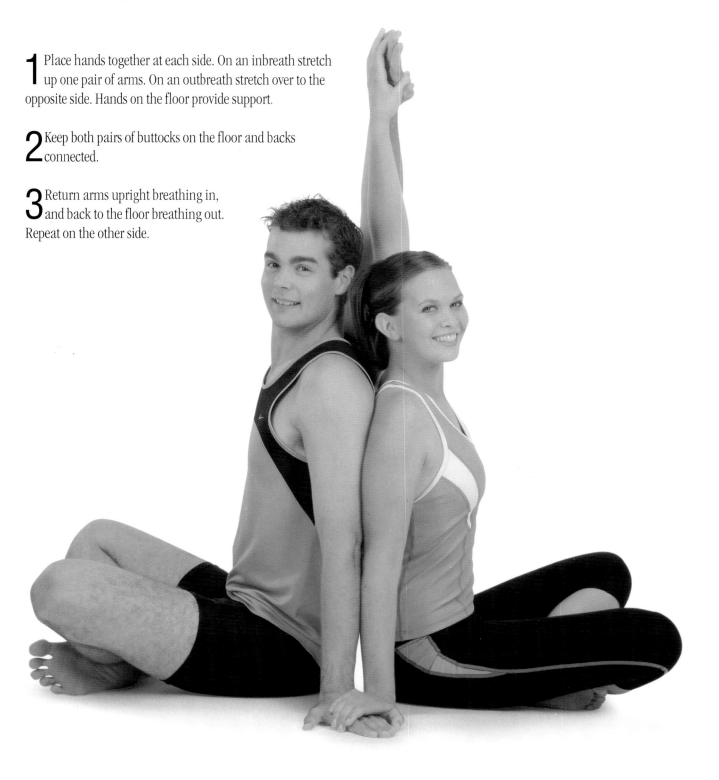

PARTNER-SHARING YOGA *(continued)*

FACING TWIST

1 Turn to face each other, legs crossed and knees touching. Each wrap your left arm behind your waist.

2 Reach forward with your right hand and take hold of your partner's left hand. Twist gently to the left and look over your left shoulder.

3 Keep buttocks firmly on the floor. Release slowly and repeat to the opposite side. (If you don't feel the stretch you could increase the distance between you and your partner's knees but proceed slowly.)

4 As in the beginning, bring hands into prayer position, look into each other's eyes. Bow slightly and thank each other for Sharing Yoga.

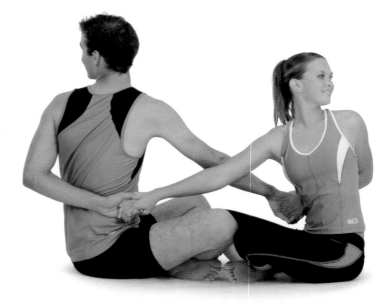

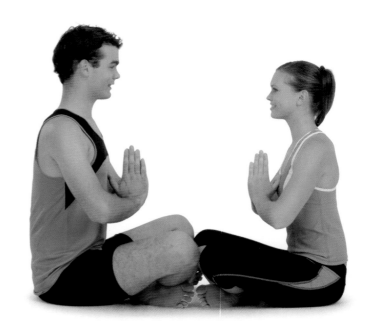

CONCLUSION

My teacher often refers to yoga as "the bridge over troubled waters". Even with the best preparation and control, there are still situations that crop up in our lives that are unpredictable and not necessarily liked.

Yoga has many facets, providing the tools to enable us to ride through the storms of life without being swamped by them. We can practise yoga for the physical benefits alone and can be very satisfied with the results.

However, yoga has the potential to be transformational if we are open to it, replacing old negative patterns with positive, life-affirming choices. I wish you all the clarity, calm and joy that I have found on this journey with yoga.

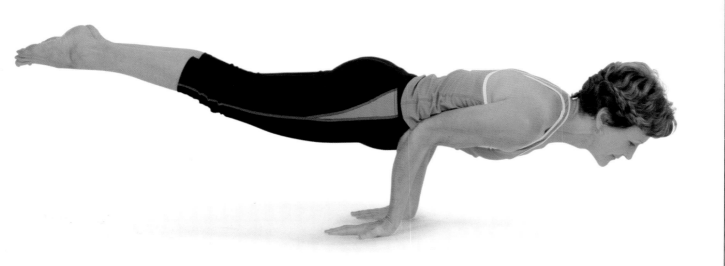

ABOUT THE AUTHOR

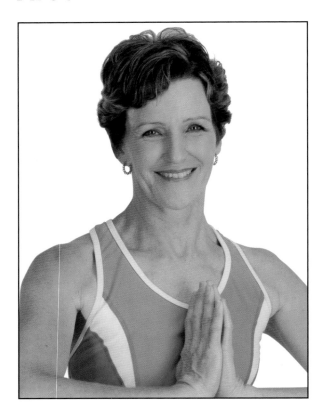

LYNLEY WOODS trained with the International Yoga Teachers' Association (IYTA) and has been teaching in the Sunshine Coast hinterland since 1997. She also instructs in the corporate sector at seminars. Considering herself an ongoing student of yoga, her teacher of 16 years is Elsa Rabold, who was a founding member of the IYTA over 30 years ago.

Elsa is a living example of the benefits of yoga – still practising and teaching at the age of 90. They are both involved in the Sunshine Coast Yoga Teachers' Network – a group of teachers dedicated to furthering the harmony and joy of yoga, as well as the knowledge and experience of its philosophy through regular retreats and workshops.

ABOUT THE MODELS

SARAH BURGESS lives on the Sunshine Coast and is currently in her second year at university, majoring in nutrition. She has been practising yoga for five years and is convinced of its contribution to a healthy lifestyle. Sarah's interests include health and travel. She feels that overall health and wellbeing will enhance the quality of her life and enable her to live to her full potential.

MATTHEW DEZOETE-BAKER lives in Brisbane and works in child care. He wants to expand this work into education and helping children. Apart from yoga, he has trained in tae kwon do and other martial arts. His interests cover a broad spectrum, from football to dancing, health and a wide range of cultural activities. His particular focus is on the Zen philosophy – the discipline of mindfulness.